Writing
Case Reports

A HOW-TO MANUAL *for* CLINICIANS

Third Edition

For physical therapists and other health care professionals
who want to contribute descriptions of practice
to their profession's body of knowledge.

Edited by Irene McEwen, PT, PhD, FAPTA

A Publication of the American Physical Therapy Association
Alexandria, Virginia

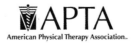

APTA
American Physical Therapy Association.

ISBN # 978-1-931369-62-6

For more information about this and other APTA publications, contact the American Physical Therapy Association, 1111 North Fairfax Street, Alexandria, VA 22314-1488, or access APTA's Online Store via APTA's Web site, www.apta.org. [Item No. C-12]

Staff Editor: Jan P Reynolds

Staff Contributors: Anita Bemis-Dougherty, PT, DPT, MAS; Gini Blodgett Birchett, MSLS; Stephen Brooks, ELS; Steven Glaros

Consultant on the *International Classification of Disability, Functioning and Health* (ICF): Diane Brandt, PTA, MS, MA

Designer and Graphic Artist: Linda Silk-Sviland

Contributors *Third Edition*

Irene McEwen, PT, PhD, FAPTA, is Ann Taylor chair in pediatrics and developmental disabilities in physical therapy and director of the postprofessional graduate program, Department of Rehabilitation Sciences, University of Oklahoma Health Sciences Center, Oklahoma City. She also is George Lynn Cross research professor and director of the Lee Mitchener Tolbert Center for Developmental Disabilities. She served as deputy editor of *Physical Therapy (PTJ)*, 2003-2005. As *PTJ*'s editor for case reports for more than 10 years, she was instrumental in developing the case report format as a way to describe physical therapist practice.

Paul Beattie, PT, PhD, OCS, is clinical associate professor, Division of Physical Therapy and Motor Control, Department of Exercise Science, University of South Carolina, Columbia.

Josh Cleland, PT, PhD, OCS, is associate professor, Physical Therapy Program, Franklin Pierce College, Concord, NH; affiliate faculty, Fellowship in Orthopaedic Manual Therapy, Regis University, Denver, Colorado; and adjunct faculty, Physical Therapy Program, Creighton University, Omaha, NE. He serves on *PTJ*'s Editorial Board.

G Kelley Fitzgerald, PT, PhD, OCS, FAPTA, is associate professor, Department of Physical Therapy, School of Health and Rehabilitation Sciences, University of Pittsburgh, and serves on *PTJ*'s Editorial Board. He is a recipient of APTA's Dorothy Briggs Memorial Scientific Inquiry Award.

Steven Z George, PT, PhD, is associate professor, Department of Physical Therapy, University of Florida, where his primary teaching responsibilities include Evidence-Based Practice I – III for the doctor of physical therapy (DPT) program. He serves on *PTJ*'s Editorial Board.

Daniel Riddle, PT, PhD, FAPTA, is Otto D Payton professor and assistant chair, Department of Physical Therapy, School of Allied Health Professions, Virginia Commonwealth University, Richmond, Virginia. He has published case reports and research reports on a variety of topics related to musculoskeletal care and serves as *PTJ*'s deputy editor in chief.

Special thanks to **Pamela Levangie, PT, PhD, FAPTA,** and **Phil McClure, PT, PhD.**

Contributors *First and Second Editions*

Irene McEwen, PT, PhD, FAPTA
Vincent Basile, PT, OCS
G Kelley Fitzgerald, PT, PhD, FAPTA
Gail M Jensen, PT, PhD, FAPTA
Daniel Riddle, PT, PhD, FAPTA
Lisa Riolo, PT, PhD, NCS

Preface to the Third Edition

More than 20 years ago, Jules Rothstein, PT, PhD, FAPTA, Editor in Chief Emeritus of *Physical Therapy* (*PTJ*), had a dream that the physical therapy profession would have a body of literature that describes practice. Back then, few case reports—as descriptions of practice—were being submitted to *PTJ*, and Jules set about to rectify that deficiency. He led an enthusiastic and focused effort not only to increase the number of case reports submitted for publication, but to ensure that published case reports describe practice with precision and scientific credibility. He wrote editorials about the need for case reports,[1-4] he gave presentations about scholarly writing at conferences around the world, he talked about case reports to anyone who would listen, and his vision of helping clinicians to write case reports of publishable quality resulted in the first edition of this book.

Jules looked forward to seeing 2 case reports in every issue of *PTJ*[4] and, thanks to his efforts, this happened before he died in 2005. Since then, *PTJ* has published even more case reports. The number of case reports in other journals also has increased, particularly in APTA section journals, such as *Journal of Neurologic Physical Therapy*, *Journal of Orthopaedic and Sports Physical Therapy*, and *Pediatric Physical Therapy*.

Jules would be pleased by the number of case reports being published, and he also would be glad to know that this manual has been a bestseller since publication of the first edition in 1996. Numerous authors have used this book to write publishable case reports, and large numbers of professional and postprofessional students have used it to fulfill the case report requirement in their education programs. Jules's dream is being realized.

When planning for the third edition, we asked people who have used the book for recommendations. The most frequent suggestions were to use more recent examples, update the chapter on searching the literature, and update the appendix containing lists of reliability and validity studies. In response to those suggestions, this edition has many new examples, and the chapter on searching the literature was rewritten. Instead of updating the appendix, however, we deleted it. We did this for several reasons. First, reliability and validity are not the only properties of tests and measures that clinicians now need to consider. Sensitivity, specificity, likelihood ratios, and minimal detectable change, for example, also need to be part of decision making and are covered in this edition. Second, the number of studies continues to increase, and any list would be out of date before the book is even published. Finally, most clinicians now have easy access to online literature databases, and a search will quickly find relevant and up-to-date research reports. In addition, with APTA's Interactive *Guide to Physical Therapist Practice* migrating to the World Wide Web, citations on reliability and validity studies for specific tests and measures will be available through that site.

Among the many other recommendations that we addressed: incorporation of the *International Classification of Functioning, Disability and Health* (ICF), *Guide to Physical Therapist Practice* terminology, and the types of focused case reports that *PTJ* now publishes.

We hope you find the third edition to be helpful. We welcome your feedback and any suggestions for materials or content related to the writing of case reports that you would like to see accessible online.

Irene R McEwen, PT, PhD, FAPTA
casereportmanual@apta.org

References

1 Rothstein JM. Clinical literature [editor's note]. *Phys Ther.* 1989;69:895-896.
2 Rothstein JM. The case for case reports. [editor's note]. *Phys Ther.* 1993;73:492-493.
3 Rothstein JM. Case reports: still a priority. [editor's note]. *Phys Ther.* 2002;82:1062-1063.
4 Rothstein JM. Rumorbusters. [editor's note]. *Phys Ther.* 2003;83:774-775.

Preface to the Second Edition

When we wrote the first edition of *Writing Case Reports: A How-to Manual for Clinicians*, we wanted it to be a user-friendly resource for clinicians. We envisioned our audience as physical therapy practitioners who had wonderful descriptions of practice to contribute to the professional literature but who needed some help in preparing a case report for publication. The increase in the number of good case reports submitted to *Physical Therapy* and other journals suggests that clinicians are responding to calls for case reports and that they are using the advice in this manual.

Perhaps an even larger audience for the manual—which we didn't anticipate—is students. *Writing Case Reports* is used as a text in many education programs that require professional and postprofessional students, residents, and fellows to write case reports as a culminating and scholarly product of their educational experiences.

Because so many education programs require the writing of case reports, we solicited input from faculty as we were planning this second edition. Many responded, and we are grateful for their input. The most common recommendation was to use terminology that is consistent with the second edition of the *Guide to Physical Therapist Practice*. The second most common recommendation was to provide more information about how to write about the diagnosis and prognosis elements of patient/client management. Several faculty members said they would like the book to include an "imperfect" manuscript of a case report for students to review, and others recommended adding a checklist of the important components of a case report. Many suggested that we update the chapter about searching for literature and the appendix that lists reliability and validity studies. We responded to all of these suggestions in this second edition.

We also tried to make the second edition more useful for occupational therapy practitioners and students. We added content from the *Guide to Occupational Therapy Practice* and included more references to case reports that have been published in the occupational therapy literature. As a faculty member of an education program that requires both physical therapist and occupational therapist students to write case reports, I look forward to using the second edition with all of my students.

Irene R McEwen, PT, PhD

Foreword to the First Edition

You're holding a dream in your hands. Almost 10 years ago, the late Dr Steve Rose—my predecessor as Editor of *Physical Therapy*—and I talked about the need for a book like this. We shared a love of physical therapy practice and wanted to see our colleagues communicating more effectively and efficiently. We longed for a public body of knowledge where ideas could be exchanged and therapists could learn from each other while revealing to the world what we do every day in our clinical settings.

Perhaps the vision that Steve and I shared was a function of our career paths. We both had spent many years in private practice before returning to school to get our doctorates and advanced training in the sciences. As a result, we never lost sight of the fact that physical therapists exist to take care of patients and clients and that there is no more important activity than high-quality patient care. We also knew that few of us were prepared to communicate about practice in a scientifically credible manner.

The vagaries of patient care are too important to be left to random communications, jargon-laden continuing education courses, or accidental dialogues. We should agree and disagree in public and grow through that discourse. We should talk to each other about what we do, and do so using clear language. We should write so that we can refine our descriptions, agree on terms and definitions, and evolve a common language of practice.

That is, we should write case reports!

Since becoming Editor of *Physical Therapy* in 1988, I have been a staunch advocate of case reports, seeking them everywhere I go. (Tony Delitto also shares the vision, and together we have made a number of presentations on writing case reports.) I have even suggested that the ability to communicate scientifically is a professional skill and that everyone graduating from a physical therapy education program should be able to write a case report. (Not everyone has agreed.)

Case reports aren't just a means by which we can all "talk shop" with each other. They are an essential part of our literature. They do not replace research reports; as you will see when you read this manual, case reports and research reports are complementary. Case reports aren't something to be taken lightly or to be published with little scrutiny. Our business is practice, and anything that describes practice must be done well. In addition, case reports provide researchers with the background they need to design outcomes studies. For these reasons, case reports, like research, must undergo peer review.

As Editor, I often am asked by authors, "Shouldn't case reports receive a less stringent review than research articles do?" Clinicians who have achieved what they believe to be exciting patient outcomes understandably want to share what they have observed. Researchers feel the same way, but they have to take part in a process that leads to refinement—the peer-review process. Taking shortcuts in this process is a lot like taking shortcuts in patient care. The results are not pretty.

I won't lie to you: Peer review isn't easy on authors. Most of us find that criticism is a lot like the flu—it is far easier and less painful to give to others than to receive it. But if you follow the guidelines in this manual, you cannot lose. Whether or not your papers are published (and odds are that they will be published if you keep trying to work out the problems), the process of writing and being reviewed is a means to professional growth. Recognize that criticism is just part of the process, and that peer review is a system in which people not only evaluate what you have done but help you make something better. Remember, too, that they are evaluating what you have done—not you, the person.

Our challenge in the coming years is to work together to establish a common body of literature. A body of literature that describes practice. A body of literature that helps new therapists know what to expect, researchers know what questions to ask, and health care managers know what we do. A body of literature that makes each of us identify with each other and understand each other better than ever before.

Thanks to the efforts of Vince Basile, Kelley Fitzgerald, Gail Jensen, Dan Riddle, Lisa Riolo, and Irene McEwen—both in her role as *Physical Therapy*'s Associate Editor for Case Reports and as this manual's editor—*Writing Case Reports* is not only a dream come true. It is a means by which even more dreams will be fulfilled for the growth of our profession.

Jules M Rothstein, PT, PhD, FAPTA (1947-2005)

TABLE OF CONTENTS

www.apta.org/crmanual
access code: giwt29wd

Real Clinicians *Do* Write Case Reports!

aybe you've developed a treatment that gets excellent results, perfected an especially useful management technique, or noted a set of similarities among certain patients that allows you to approach those patients in a unique and effective way. You describe your idea to a few colleagues, and they express interest and enthusiasm. You present it at an informal meeting or an in-service program, and again the feedback is positive. Then, just as you've begun to enjoy that warm glow of satisfaction, someone utters the dreaded words:

"You really ought to write that up for a journal."

Suddenly, there isn't enough air in the room. You think about how much you enjoy direct patient contact. "Real" clinicians, you say to yourself, spend their time treating patients, not writing.

For most of us, "putting it down on paper" ranks among our biggest fears. The feeling of competence we have in the clinic or the classroom fades when we are faced with the great unknown of writing for publication. We remember stories of colleagues who submitted articles to journals and were "savaged" by the editorial review process. We fear that if we write, the same thing will happen to us. We also fear that if our ideas are actually published, we will be exposing ourselves to criticism. What's the result of this collective phobia? A profession that fails to share basic information—the kind of information required to develop the concepts, methods, and proofs that can improve patient care, help justify our treatments to payers, and distinguish us from faith healers and faddists.

The irony is that we clinicians consider ourselves to be the Great Practical Communicators. Talk with any group of us, and you immediately strike a vein of common concern for communication

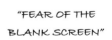

"FEAR OF THE
BLANK SCREEN"

and teaching. And we do communicate effectively—even passionately—on a one-to-one, day-to-day basis. But we still fail to share information effectively. We consider documentation to be a routine aspect of practice, but we don't take the next step to expand that documentation to its logical conclusion: writing a case report for publication in the peer-reviewed literature, where it can become a part of the professional body of knowledge.

You might not realize it, but you already have many of the skills required to write successful case reports. All you need is a practical tool to help you refine and apply those skills. This how-to manual was designed to do just that.

If you're a professional or postprofessional student, this book also is for you. Many education programs now require students to write case reports, which is an excellent way for students to demonstrate their clinical decision-making abilities related to a real patient. Even if you think a case report is only an academic exercise and you don't plan to submit it for publication, you might surprise yourself. Students have written many published case reports, and faculty members often are happy to help students prepare and submit them for publication.

Reading this book isn't like reading a novel; you don't have to begin at the beginning. But you might find it helpful to do so, especially if you have limited experience in writing case reports. Part I shows you how to prepare for writing a case report; Part II takes you through the writing process and explains peer review. For readers who want more details, Appendixes contain "case report checklists" that will help you keep track as you write your report. With this edition, we have added supplements that manual purchasers can access online only: **eAppendix 1**, "Annotations for Published Case Reports," which shows how authors dealt with components of the case report; **eAppendix 2**, "Fictional Case Report," which highlights aspects of clinical decision making that can be described in case reports; and **eAppendix 3**, "What Peer Review Feedback Looks Like," which provides composite examples of constructive reviewer comments on case reports.

Whether you decide to work on your own or with others, the writing process will offer you many opportunities. You'll be able to examine your own clinical observations and reasoning, share your work with a larger audience, give something back to a profession that is so much a part of you—and ultimately do what all "real" clinicians want to do: improve patient care.

Good luck!

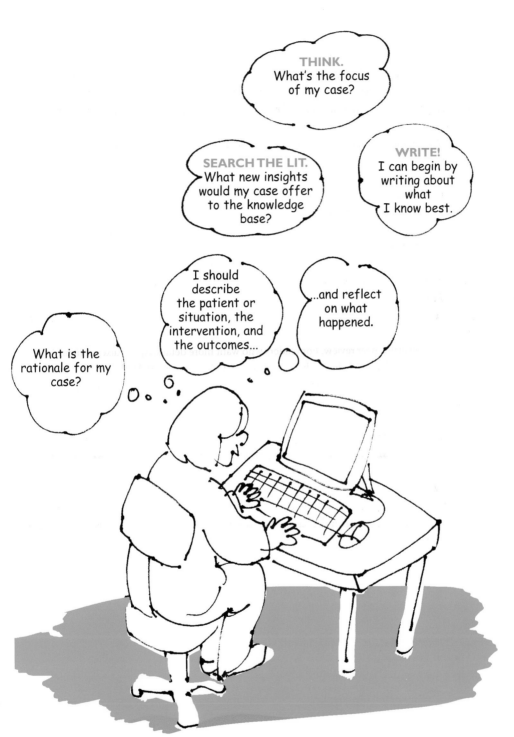

The Case Report Writing Process

PART I

Before You Write

"The whole of science is nothing more than a refinement of everyday thinking."

Albert Einstein

Why Write Case Reports?

Case reports can't prove effectiveness—
but they can lead researchers to do the
kinds of studies that will.

ase reports look a lot like research reports. They have a title, an abstract, and an introduction that reviews related literature to provide rationale for the management of the case. They also have a case description that provides information about the patient (or other entity) and the intervention, a section on outcomes, and a discussion. These components are covered in detail later on.

Although case reports *look* a lot like research reports, they aren't. Unlike randomized controlled trials and other experimental studies, case reports are solely descriptions of practice. They can't test hypotheses or establish cause and effect, and the outcomes that they report can't be generalized to other patients or entities. Experimental designs (Table 1) have the controls that allow identification of cause-and-effect relationships between the independent variable (the intervention) and the dependent variable (the observed response or result). Lacking such controls, case reports can be viewed as "pre-experimental." So, why write them? Because they generate ideas, hypotheses, and techniques that can be tested or studied later through controlled experiments.[1,2]

Physical Therapy (*PTJ*) alone has published hundreds of case reports since 1980, with more than half published since the first edition of this book was released. The number of published clinical trials, which can provide evidence for practice, has increased as well. But

TABLE 1. Categories of Scientific Inquiry

Experimental Designs

The structure of experimental designs allows researchers to identify cause-and-effect relationships between independent and dependent variables. The strength of the evidence depends on the characteristics of the design, which fall into these classic categories[a]:

True experimental design	Participants are randomly assigned to experimental and control or comparison groups. Provides the strongest evidence of cause-and-effect relationships.
Quasi-experimental design	Lacks random assignment of participants, a control or comparison group, or both. Often used in clinical research when researchers study already existing groups, when random assignment is not possible, or both.
Single-subject design	A type of quasi-experimental design that lacks the generalizability of group designs. There are many different types of single-subject designs, all of which are characterized by repeated measurements of the dependent variable.

Nonexperimental Designs

Nonexperimental designs do not manipulate the independent variable and cannot determine cause-and-effect relationships. There are 3 general types[b]:

Descriptive research	Discloses existing conditions or examines relationships among variables, using such means as direct observation, surveys, and interviews. Includes correlational studies; qualitative studies; case studies[c]; investigations to identify normative values or developmental patterns; and epidemiological studies, such as cohort and case-control studies, which describe and predict health risks.
Evaluation research	Assesses how well a program or a policy is meeting its goals and objectives. Can provide a means to document quality of care and program effectiveness or efficiency.
Methodological research	Involves the development of measurement tools and the assessment of their psychometric properties and their usefulness in answering clinical questions.

Case Reports

Case reports describe practice. Their credibility is enhanced by attempting to control, rule out, or acknowledge alternative explanations for outcomes, but case reports do not impose the types of controls required to identify cause-and-effect relationships among variables. Case reports often focus on a patient or a group of patients (no more than 10), but they also may focus on institutions, facilities, education programs, or other definable units. Topics can include patient/client management, ethical dilemmas, use of equipment or devices, or administrative or educational concerns.

[a] Campbell D, Stanley J. *Experimental and Quasi-Experimental Designs for Research.* Chicago, IL: Rand McNally; 1963.

[b] Portney LG, Watkins MP. *Foundations of Clinical Research: Applications to Practice.* 3rd ed. Upper Saddle River, NJ: Prentice Hall; 2009.

[c] "Case study" refers to a type of research methodology that has its own procedures and standards and is distinct from case reports.

anyone who has searched for evidence to make clinical decisions knows that many gaps remain in the scientific literature. Case reports can help to fill those gaps. And, there *always* will be a need to describe the process of clinical decision making and the details of patient/client management —something that case reports are ideally designed to do.

A case report can serve more than one purpose. It might convey experiences to other clinicians while revealing hypotheses for future research, or it might provide material for teaching and learning while assisting in the evolution of theory. It might persuade or motivate other practitioners, or help develop practice guidelines and critical pathways.

Share Clinical Experiences

Whether you function primarily as a clinician, an administrator, an educator, or a researcher, you spend most of your professional life asking questions. Clinicians ask such questions as: How often should a 2-year-old child with spastic diplegia receive what type of intervention to accomplish which goals? How does the examination and evaluation lead to determining the diagnosis and prognosis for a 45-year-old man following severe hand trauma? What approaches can be used to measure and increase physical therapist students' responsibility for learning? What independent and dependent variables are most likely to provide useful information in a study of intervention for conditions related to stroke in patients with certain characteristics?

It isn't easy to find answers to these and the countless other questions that are asked in clinics, classrooms, and laboratories every day. Research articles, textbooks, continuing education courses, Web sites, and other sources of information can contribute to our knowledge base; however, these sources are likely to provide only partial answers—and they might not wrestle with how to make those answers work in the real world.

Case reports are better than sharing experiences through conversation—when published in a peer-reviewed journal, the case report represents the consensus of a small panel of experts.

The very nature of the case report requires the kind of details that would be necessary for another clinician to implement the approach or intervention discussed in the report. Alnwick,[3] for example, described his experience with a patient referred for physical therapy with a diagnosis of fibromyalgia. He began with a detailed account of the patient's history, symptoms, and diagnoses over the 4 years prior to referral to his clinic. He then clearly described his examination and evaluation, which led him to refer the patient back to her primary care physician, with a recommendation for referral to a neurologist. Alnwick suspected that the patient had serotonin syndrome, which the neurologist later diagnosed. Alnwick's clear, detailed descriptions of examination, evaluation, and clinical reasoning provide a wealth of information for clinicians who have similar patients. Such information rarely is provided in research reports or even in textbooks, continuing education courses, or Web sites.

Patients' desired outcomes are considered as part of the research process more often today than in the past,[4] but they must be identified and addressed directly every day in practice. As a component of their examination, Riddle and colleagues[5] determined and reported the goal that their patient with low back pain wanted to accomplish. They described their decision making as they worked their way through the Hypothesis-Oriented Algorithm for Clinicians (HOAC II)[6] to design, implement, evaluate, and modify the intervention. Each step of their decision-making

Supply enough details
so colleagues can
replicate what you did

process could offer information or inspiration for other clinicians managing patients with similar conditions.

Sharing experiences through case reports is similar to sharing experiences through conversation with colleagues. Ideas are stimulated; new insights are provided. There are 2 important differences, however. First, the case report provides sufficient detail to allow colleagues who are not involved in the conversation to replicate the clinical reasoning process. Second, a case report published in a peer-reviewed journal represents the consensus of a small panel of experts. No, case reports cannot give definitive answers about effectiveness of interventions or the validity of a hypothesis, but they do allow readers to benefit not only from the experiences of the authors but also from the knowledge of the reviewers, whether those reviewers are manuscript reviewers, course instructors, or colleagues.

Illustrate Evidence-Based Practice

What does "evidence-based practice" really mean? Does it mean that all patient/client management decisions have to be based on research? Does it mean that if evidence doesn't exist, clinicians should do nothing until it *does* exist? Does "evidence-based" mean that clinicians are free to continue to do what they've always done even if research evidence isn't available? The answer to all of these questions is "**no**"!

The most widely used definition of *evidence-based practice* (really of "evidence-based medicine," which started it all) comes from Straus and colleagues: "The integration of best research evidence with our clinical expertise and our patient's unique values and circumstances."[7(p1)] When these 3 elements are integrated, "clinicians and patients form a diagnostic and therapeutic alliance which optimizes clinical outcomes and quality of life."[8(p1)] Remember, "evidence-based practice means using the best possible data to make a decision— not to justify a decision that's already been made."[9(p7)]

Although evidence hierarchies[7] place case reports at or near the bottom, according to Jenicek, case reports "often remain the 'first line of evidence.' This is where everything begins."[10] Case reports are an ideal mechanism to illustrate how clinicians integrate the best available research evidence, clinical expertise, and patient choice. Parker[11] wrote a case report that illustrates the process of providing care based on research evidence. The patient was an older woman with a fractured femur, and the author needed to decide on medical and surgical management. At the beginning of the report, Parker defined a limit of spending no more than 4 hours on an office computer to identify the evidence. The report first described the computerized databases that Parker explored and the types of articles that the author read (reviews of randomized trials, when available). The report then described the evidence found for decision making about initial management; whether to operate, and, if so, when and what implant to use; anticoagulation prophylaxis; postoperative care and rehabilitation; and prevention of further fractures.

Evidence-based practice combines the best available research evidence, clinical expertise, and patient values. Case reports are an excellent way to integrate these elements.

The rehabilitation portion of Parker's case report is limited and basically concluded that discharge to home and "community services" may be beneficial. Imagine the contributions that case reports about evidence-based rehabilitation for this and other types of patients would make to the literature! **Chapter 3** provides helpful information about how to search the literature to find evidence to support your patient/client management decisions.

Develop Hypotheses for Research

Case reports can make an important contribution to the process of scientific inquiry by providing a broad base of descriptive information that researchers can test empirically.[1,2] The level and type of description that case reports provide usually are not possible in research investigations that examine a limited number of variables under controlled conditions. Each detail of a case report has the potential to become a variable for future research that in turn could help provide definitive answers to questions about practice.[12] If research is to answer the questions that practitioners are asking in the clinic, the generating of ideas cannot be left solely to the researcher's imagination.

In his "defense of case reports and case series," Vandenbroucke gave an example of a systematic review of case reports and case series of ischemic colitis among young people, which led to the hypothesis that "it seemed to be a disease of young women, elicited by oral contraceptives in particular."[13(p332)] This hypothesis was later supported by a case–control study.[14]

Deutsch et al[15] showed how case reports can help identify research variables and hypotheses in rehabilitation. The authors described the feasibility of using a commercially available gaming system as part of training for visual-perceptual processing, postural control, and functional mobility in an adolescent with spastic diplegic cerebral palsy in a school-based setting. They noted positive outcomes in impairments, activities, and participation, and, although a case report can't determine cause and effect, they were able to identify several hypotheses that they hoped would be "the springboard for additional research."[15(p1196)] One of the hypotheses was that combining training for visual-perceptual processing, postural control, and endurance might improve functional mobility.

Build Problem-Solving Skills

Case reports are used extensively in the academic programs of such professions as business and law to help students develop critical-thinking and problem-solving skills. Academicians in these fields promote the "case study method," that is, the use of real or fictional cases that provide opportunities to become familiar with a variety of facts and practices, to identify critical problems and issues, to make decisions, to devise courses of action, and to explore possible outcomes and alternatives.[16,17] Because these are the same skills that professional physical therapist education programs strive to develop in their students, case reports could be of similar value in professional education courses. A greater number and variety of case reports must be published, however, before this purpose can be served.

Another valuable learning experience for students—and for practitioners—is the process of writing a case report.[18,19] During the search for literature to support the case report, not only does the writer gain knowledge directly related to the topic, but the process of locating and synthesizing related information to justify or question a procedure can be even more informative. Students and clinicians who have had little experience in reviewing the literature may be astounded to find scant support for even the most common of clinical procedures—a valuable lesson in itself.

Learning continues as the writer describes each step in patient/client management. To be understood by the reader, these descriptions must be clear, complete, jargon-free, and justified—which requires the writer to identify all of the relevant details and reveal the decision-making process. Such opportunities for inspection of our own individual practice are rare in the midst of most practitioners' and students' day-to-day responsibilities. Just as educational is the process of reflection. Reflection is required to write the discussion section, which shows how a case illuminates what is known about the clinical problem and how the case relates to other literature.[20]

> Opportunities for this kind of inspection of your own practice are rare in the midst of day-to-day responsibilities.

Perhaps the most valuable learning experience comes from submitting the case report for publication. Although the peer-review process may seem intimidating at first, writers should remember that it is designed to help them communicate their ideas as effectively and as credibly as possible. If the writer thoughtfully answers the reviewers' questions and carefully considers their suggestions, the writer, the literature, and the profession will be enlightened. **Chapter 11** covers the peer-review process.

Support, Enhance, or Cast Doubt on Theory Underlying Practice

Theory can be described as a body of related knowledge that serves as a framework for organizing complex and diverse information. Such a framework allows us to fit fragments of information into a larger picture and to predict beyond what we personally have experienced.

Theories are never finished. They are continually expanded and modified to accommodate new information that supports or refutes the theoretical constructs. Some theories encompass a large body of knowledge; others have a much more narrow scope. Dynamic systems theory—discussed by Heriza[21] in the context of movement, for example—is so broad that it has application to such diverse phenomena as weather forecasting and infant development. Other theories, such as the convex-concave theory of arthrokinematic motion,[22] are much more focused.

How can case reports support or enhance theory? By providing real-life examples of a theory's application, or, as Lazarus and Davison[23] described it, by putting "the 'meat' on the theoretical skeleton." This meat is especially important for broad theories that can be difficult to apply in practice. Many clinicians would eagerly read case reports that describe application of motor learning theory to management of a child with cerebral palsy or application of dynamic systems theory to management of a patient with arthritis. Case reports also can enhance theory by describing experiences that go beyond current theory and can suggest hypotheses that could be tested by researchers to advance the theoretical framework.

> Case reports can put "the 'meat' on the theoretical skeleton," describing the application of theory, such as the application of motor learning theory to management of a child with cerebral palsy.

Sometimes case reports cast doubt on theory. In a case report about a patient with limited shoulder motion, McClure and Flowers[24] challenged the convex-concave theory of arthrokinematic movement by reviewing literature to support their contention that humeral translation may be a function of tension in capsular tissues rather than of joint surface geometry. This challenge could easily lead to a debate about the causes of shoulder motion limitation and raise questions for future investigations.

Persuade and Motivate

Almost every health care profession has experienced drastic change in recent years. Rehabilitation practices certainly are very different from what they were, due to events both within and outside the rehabilitation professions. III STEP: Linking Movement Science and Intervention—a conference cosponsored in 2005 by the American Physical Therapy Association's (APTA) Section on Pediatrics and Neurology Section—is an example of an internal event that had a major impact on physical therapist practice. The conference and the series of articles based on conference presentations published in *PTJ*[25] introduced the *International Classification of Functioning, Disability and Health* (ICF)[26] to many clinicians and researchers. These presentations and articles also caused many physical therapists to view neural plasticity and intensity of practice very differently from the way they viewed them prior to the conference. Health care reform efforts initiated during the 1990s are examples of external events; in a relatively short period of time, they had a major impact on the way in which we practice, teach, and conduct research.

> Help colleagues deal with change

Resistance to change is natural, particularly when we are comfortable with the way we have "always done things" and when we are not certain what to do instead. Case reports give how-to-do-it examples, and, because they are story-like and transparently applicable, they can be an appealing way to begin the change process. Schreiber[27] gave an example of increased frequency of physical therapy for a 2 ½-year-old child with a chromosomal abnormality. He described the decision-making process associated with increasing the frequency from once every 2 weeks to 4 times per week for 4 weeks. The child's motor skills improved more rapidly over the 4-week period than they had prior to the increased frequency. This case report and others like it could help persuade clinicians to try a period of increased frequency of intervention and also could help persuade early intervention program administrators and third-party payers to agree to increased frequency—as long as meaningful outcomes are identified, measured, and documented.

Another change for many clinicians has been the need to consider context when applying the ICF. Context has long been an important factor in occupational therapy, which Head and Patterson[28] illustrated in their case report of a 79-year-old man with a variety of health-related problems that limited his activities and restricted his participation. The case report compared examination and evaluation in the clinic setting with examination and evaluation in his home— and highlighted the value of evaluation and intervention within the context of the natural, home environment. This case report could help other clinicians to see the importance of context and could promote an increase in service delivery in patients' natural environments.

Case reports also might help persuade administrators to agree to clinicians' proposals for organizational change. A case report, for example, might clearly illustrate the implementation of an electronic documentation system to reduce costs, improve patient care, and collect outcomes data. Case reports giving real-life solutions to common professional education problems also could inspire change. Faculty might be persuaded to try innovative ways to select students for admission, provide clinical education, schedule laboratory sessions for large numbers of students, or improve students' professional writing skills.

Help Develop Guidelines and Pathways

Because our health care environment has become increasingly complex, practitioners, academicians, researchers, third-party payers, and policymakers must determine with greater accuracy what works for whom and how long it takes.[29] Success (and even professional survival) depends on the accuracy of patient/client management predictions—and currently there is little research on which to base these decisions. Again, case reports cannot provide definitive answers about effectiveness, but the descriptions of clinical practice that they provide can be a rich source of experience (eg, observations of the natural history of conditions and suggestions about the ways in which patients can be classified) that can contribute to the development of practice guidelines, critical pathways, and other patient/client management approaches.

> Case reports can help practitioners deal with change, influence administrators, and persuade physicians and insurers of the value of services for particular patients.

Three documents on patient/client management that are important for rehabilitation professionals are APTA's *Guide to Physical Therapist Practice*[30] and the American Occupational Therapy Association's (AOTA) *Guide to Occupational Therapy Practice*[31] and *Occupational Therapy Practice Framework: Domain and Process*.[32] Primary purposes of these documents include improvement of quality of care and reduction of costs. Case reports that provide information pertinent to the natural history of various conditions and to diagnostic classification, prognosis, and intervention have contributed and will continue to contribute to the development and revision of these association documents.

Case reports also can be used to help identify and reduce variations in practice. Although research is required to establish cause-and-effect relationships, information from an accumulation of case reports can be useful for the purposes of comparison. If the patient outcomes described by case reports seem to be superior to outcomes in a clinic, a closer look at the approaches used in the clinic may be warranted. The clinicians might consider implementing approaches that the case reports suggest could be more effective.

> Case reports can provide critical information about patient/client management and practice variation.

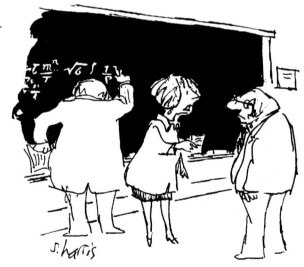

"WE COLLABORATE. 'M AN EXPERT, BUT NOT AN AUTHORITY, AND DR. GELPAS S AN AUTHORITY, BUT NOT AN EXPERT"

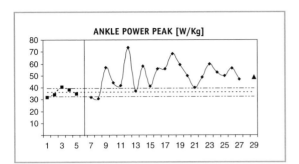

FIGURE 1. Unlike case reports, single-subject studies use experimental controls and repeated measures and, therefore, can show cause-and-effect relationships among variables. This figure shows the baseline measurements of the ankle power peak of a patient with chronic stroke and his ankle power peak after intervention that consisted of electromyographic biofeedback and application of motor learning principles. By repeatedly measuring ankle power prior to and after intervention, the researchers attempted to control for rival explanations and show that the intervention caused the increase in ankle power.

Reprinted with permission of American Society of Neurorehabilitation from Jonsdottir J, Cattaneo D, Regola A, et al. Concepts of motor learning applied to a rehabilitation protocol using biofeedback to improve gait in a chronic stroke patient: an A-B system study with multiple gait analyses. *Neurorehabilitation & Neural Repair.* 2007;21:190-194.

Case Reports Versus Case Studies and Single-Subject Designs

The terms "case report" and "case study" sometimes are used interchangeably, and their definitions tend to overlap. For the purposes of this manual, "case report" refers to descriptions of practice that do not involve research methods. A "case study," which may be similar in appearance to a case report, refers to a type of research methodology and has procedures and standards of its own; it is included as a type of "descriptive research" in Table 1. Schmoll[33] and Merriam[34] included the case study as one of the major types of research designs in qualitative research, whereas other authors have described case studies as yielding both qualitative and quantitative data that can be used to explore, describe, or predict various phenomena.[29] Prior to 1996, *PTJ* sometimes published case reports in which authors referred to their work as "case studies" or "studies." *PTJ* now reserves the terms "case study" and "study" for types of research reports.

Case reports also have been confused with single-subject designs. Unlike case reports, single-subject studies use experimental controls and repeated measurements to show cause-and-effect relationships among variables. Jonsdottir and colleagues[35] used an A-B type of single-subject design to demonstrate that electromyographic feedback combined with application of motor learning principles (the independent variables) improved ankle power at push-off and gait parameters in a patient with chronic hemiplegia. Figure 1 shows the baseline (A phase, to the left of the vertical line) and intervention (B phase, to the right of the vertical line) measurements for ankle power at push-off. The researchers took 5 baseline measurements over a 2-week period before starting the intervention. The baseline data were somewhat variable but stable, indicating that the patient's ankle power did not change over the 2-week period. Following the baseline measurements, the authors started the intervention, which the patient received 3 times per week for a total of 20 sessions. They measured ankle power approximately 2 hours after each session and the day after the last session. (The graph shows the 21 B phase measurements to the right of the baseline measurements.) Six weeks later, they measured power again to assess carryover, which is indicated on the graph by the triangle, the last data point.

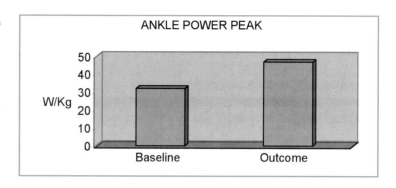

FIGURE 2. If Jonsdottir et al[6] had written a case report, these are data that they might have collected. Again, as with an A-B design, variables other than the intervention could have caused or contributed to the outcomes.

In this single-subject study, the researchers used the 2-standard-deviation bandwidth method to analyze differences between the phases. The middle horizontal line on the graph indicates the mean of the baseline measurements, and the upper and lower lines indicate 2 standard deviations above and below the baseline mean. Because at least 2 consecutive data points during the intervention phase were above the upper horizontal line, ankle power was considered to be significantly greater during the intervention phase.

An A-B design is a weak type of single-subject design because something other than the intervention might have occurred to improve the outcome (in this instance, ankle power). For example, after the intervention was initiated, the patient might have started an exercise program without informing the researchers. Other types of single-subject designs are stronger, such as multiple baseline, withdrawal, and alternating treatment designs.[1]

Case reports are much like an A-B single-subject design, except that outcome measurements are not taken as repeatedly or as systematically as they are for an A-B design. Case reports often have only one preintervention measurement and one postintervention measurement—which is what usually happens in practice. Some authors, however, may report intermediate measurement data. **Figure 2** shows the data that Jonsdottir et al[35] might have collected if they had written a case report. Again, as with an A-B design, variables other than the intervention could have caused or contributed to the outcomes.

Although the purpose of a case report is to describe practice, not to determine cause and effect, some features of the A-B design are useful for case reports. Kazdin[2] suggested several ways to strengthen the credibility of case reports and make them similar to an A-B design:

1) Systematically collect reliable data.

2) Take several measurements over time, before and after the intervention.

3) Use interventions with strong, immediate effects.

4) Report application of the intervention with several patients (or other entities, depending on the focus of your report).

Chapter 1: Why Write Case Reports?

The Value of Reporting Nonpatient Cases

Because the preponderance of published case reports involves patients, this manual focuses on patient-related case reports. But case reports that do not involve patients or that involve patients only peripherally also can make a valuable contribution to the professional knowledge base.

A case report can describe or demonstrate the development and implementation of a new administrative or educational process or modifications to existing approaches to address special problems or needs. In these cases, the detail is concentrated in the rationale for the new or modified process, in the steps taken to develop the process, and in the direct application and evaluation of the process in the context of the intended target population and the setting in which the process would be used.

In a case report that could be of value to educators, Low[36] wrote about **the use of online technology with physical therapist students during their internships.** The introduction of the report described the need to support students' learning and critical thinking skills during their internships away from campus and the potential value of an online education program. The report then described the students involved and the development and implementation of an education program using Web-based courseware. Following their internships, students who were and were not involved in the online program evaluated their critical thinking skills, and the group involved in the online program evaluated their online experience. The outcomes of the evaluation and the descriptions of the online program give information that would be useful for other education programs looking for ways to promote student learning and critical thinking skills during internships. The case report also is a good example of the type of contribution that educators who are not researchers can make to the literature of their professions.

> Almost any aspect of practice is a potential topic for a case report.

Another education-related case report that could be helpful for educators discussed **accommodations for a physical therapist student with activity limitations and participation restrictions.**[37] The report reviewed legislation related to accommodation for people with disabilities and literature on accommodation in education programs. The case description section described the student and her limitations, the process for seeking accommodation, and the variety of accommodations that the program put in place. The outcome was that the student graduated, passed the licensure examination, and became employed in an outpatient clinic with minimal assistance from physical therapist assistants and aides. This case report shares useful information with other educators about legal requirements for accommodation, the process for obtaining accommodation, and specific accommodations that allowed a student to complete a physical therapist education program and become successfully employed.

In a case report on **patient-related equipment and procedures in telerehabilitation for people with neurologic conditions,**[38] Savard and colleagues first described the **challenge of obtaining specialty health care services** when people live in unserved or underserved communities and the **technologies that can help provide services from a distance.** The authors then explained their use of videoconferencing for rehabilitation specialty consultation, including physical therapist consultation, for people with neurologic conditions living in rural Minnesota and American Samoa. Outcomes included the number of patients and their characteristics, the changes in rehabilitation care following consultation, results of patient and local clinician surveys, and mileage saved. The report then went on to give detailed case examples of an adult and a child involved in the telerehabilitation program, and the discussion section provided useful, specific recommendations for others planning similar programs.

Faculty development was the topic of another useful nonpatient case report. Peterson and Umphred[39] described the need for faculty scholarship to meet accreditation standards. They then explained the **development and implementation of a Scholarly Activity Plan for faculty**. One outcome: achievement of the short-term goal to meet accreditation standards. Faculty scholarship is a "hot" topic in many physical therapist education programs, so imagine the value of more case reports that describe programs' attempts to define and increase scholarship among faculty.

Two other case reports dealt with administrative concerns. One reviewed and recommended **guidelines for e-mail communication** in psychiatric practice and gave case examples of the issues involved.[40] Another case report described **modification of an evidence-based practice course** for occupational therapist students for application in a clinic as a strategy to promote evidence-based practice among clinicians.[41]

As you can see, almost any aspect of practice is a potential topic for a case report. Administrators, academic and clinical educators, clinicians, and students all have experiences to share that could be useful to others.

NEXT

What Kind of Case Do You Have in Mind?
It's worth saying one more time: Case reports cannot identify cause-and-effect relationships between interventions and outcomes. They do, however, give us meticulous descriptions of practice that make important contributions to the professional literature. The first key to success in writing case reports is to choose your case wisely.

Chapter 1: Why Write Case Reports?

References

1 Barlow DH, Hersen M. *Single Case Experimental Designs*. 2nd ed. New York, NY: Pergamon Press; 1984.

2 Kazdin AE. Drawing valid inferences from case studies. *Journal of Counseling and Clinical Psychology*. 1981;19:183-192.

3 Alnwick GM. Misdiagnosis of serotonin syndrome as fibromyalgia and the role of physical therapists. *Phys Ther*. 2008;88:757-765.

4 Teram E, Schachter CL, Stalker CA. The case for integrating grounded theory and participatory action research: empowering clients to inform professional practice. *Qual Health Res*. 2005;15:1129-1140.

5 Riddle DL, Rothstein JM, Echternach JL. Application of the HOAC II: an episode of care for a patient with low back pain. *Phys Ther*. 2003;83:471-485.

6 Rothstein JM, Echternach JL, Riddle DL. The Hypothesis-Oriented Algorithm for Clinicians II (HOAC II): a guide for patient management. *Phys Ther*. 2003;83:455-470.

7 Straus SE, Richardson WS, Glasziou P, Haynes RB. *Evidence-Based Medicine: How to Practice and Teach EBM*. 3rd ed. New York, NY: Churchill Livingstone Inc; 2005.

8 Sackett DL, Straus SE, Richardson WS, et al. *Evidence-Based Medicine: How to Practice and Teach EBM*. 2nd ed. New York, NY: Churchill Livingstone Inc; 2000.

9 Rothstein JM. Thirty years later...[editor's note]. *Phys Ther*. 2000;80:6-7.

10 Jenicek M. *Clinical Case Reporting in Evidence-Based Medicine*. Oxford, United Kingdom: Butterworth-Heinemann; 1999:117.

11 Parker MJ. Managing an elderly patient with a fractured femur. *Br Med J*. 2000;320:102-103.

12 McEwen IR, Karlan GR. Case studies: why and how. *Augment Altern Commun*. 1990;6:69-75.

13 Vandenbroucke JP. In defense of case reports and case series. *Ann Intern Med*. 2001;134:330-334.

14 Deana DG, Dean PJ. Reversible ischemic colitis in young women: association with oral contraceptive use. *Am J Surg Pathol*. 1995;19:454-462.

15 Deutsch JE, Borbely M, Filler J,et al. Use of a low-cost, commercially available gaming console (Wii) for rehabilitation of an adolescent with cerebral palsy. *Phys Ther*. 2008;88:1196-1207.

16 Henson KT. Case study in teacher education. *The Educational Forum*. 1988;52:236-241.

17 Ready RK. The case study II [letter to the editor]. *J Appl Behav Sci*. 1968;4:232-235.

18 DeBakey L, DeBakey S. The case report, I: guidelines for preparation. *Int J Cardiol*. 1983;4:357-364.

19 Petrusa ER, Weiss GB. Writing case reports: an educationally valuable experience for house officers. *J Med Educ*. 1982;57:415-417.

20 Roland CG. The case report. *JAMA*. 1968;205:83-84.

21 Heriza CB. Implications of a dynamical systems approach to understanding infant kicking behavior. *Phys Ther*. 1991;71:222-235.

22 Kaltenborn FM. *Mobilization of the Extremity Joints*. Oslo, Norway: Olaf Norlis Bokhandel Universitetsgaten; 1980.

23 Lazarus AA, Davison GC. Clinical innovation in research and practice. In: Bergin AE, Garfield SL, eds. *Handbook of Psychotherapy and Behavior Change: An Empirical Analysis*. New York, NY: John Wiley & Sons Inc; 1971:196-213.

24 McClure PW, Flowers KR. Treatment of limited shoulder motion: a case study based on biomechanical considerations. *Phys Ther*. 1992;72:929-936.

25 III STEP series. Available at: http://www.ptjournal.org/collections/. Accessed December 1, 2008.

26 World Health Organization. *International Classification of Functioning, Disability and Health*; 2001. Available at: http://www.who.int/classifications/icf/en/. Accessed December 1, 2008.

27 Schreiber J. Increased intensity of physical therapy for a child with gross motor developmental delay: a case report. *Physical & Occupational Therapy in Pediatrics*. 2004;24(4):63-78.

28 Head J, Patterson V. Performance context and its role in treatment planning. *Am J Occup Ther*. 1997;51:453-457.

29 DePoy D, Gitlin LN. *Introduction to Research: Multiple Strategies for Health and Human Services*. St Louis, Mo: CV Mosby Co; 1994.

30 *Guide to Physical Therapist Practice*. Rev 2nd ed. Alexandria, VA: American Physical Therapy Association; 2003.

31 Moyers PA, Dale LM. *Guide to Occupational Therapy Practice*. 2nd ed. Bethesda, MD: American Occupational Therapy Association; 2007

32 *Occupational Therapy Practice Framework: Domain and Process*, ed 2. *Am J Occup Ther*. 2008;62:625–683.

33 Schmoll BJ. Qualitative research. In: Bork CE, ed. *Research in Physical Therapy*. Philadelphia, Pa: JB Lippincott Co; 1993:83-124.

34 Merriam S. *Case Study Research in Education: A Qualitative Approach*. San Francisco, CA: Jossey-Bass Inc Publishers; 1988.

35 Jonsdottir J, Cattaneo D, Regola A, et al. Concepts of motor learning applied to a rehabilitation protocol using biofeedback to improve gait in a chronic stroke patient: an A-B system study with multiple gait analyses. *Neurorehabilitation & Neural Repair.* 2007;21: 190-194.

36 Low S. Supporting student learning during physical therapist student internships using online technology. *Journal of Physical Therapy Education.* 2008;22(1):75-82.

37 Francis NJ, Salzman A, Polomsky D, Huffman E. Accommodations for a student with a physical disability in a professional physical therapist education program. *Journal of Physical Therapy Education.* 2007;21(2):60-65.

38 Savard L, Borstad A, Tkachuck J, et al. Telerehabilitation consultations for clients with neurologic diagnoses: cases from rural Minnesota and American Samoa. *Neurorehabilitation.* 2003;18:93-102.

39 Peterson CA, Umphred DA. A structured faculty development process for scholarship in young faculty: a case report. *Journal of Physical Therapy Education.* 2005;19(3):86-88.

40 Silk KR, Yager J. Suggested guidelines for e-mail communication in psychiatric practice. *J Clin Psychiatry.* 2003;64:799-806.

41 Bailey DM, Bornstein J, Ryan S. A case report of evidence-based practice: from academia to clinic. *Am J Occup Ther.* 2007;61:85-91.

CHAPTER 2

Choosing a Case, or Cases, to Report

Your case does not have to be unusual or unique to contribute to the body of knowledge.

Cases do not always have to be unusual or unique to be published in *PTJ* or in many other journals. Some medical journals are interested in publishing reports only of new phenomena or new approaches to diagnosis and intervention,[1,2] but that's probably because some areas of medicine are much older and have a large cache of case reports and other professional literature from which to draw. *Annals of Internal Medicine* publishes a category of article called "Clinical Observations," which includes case reports of "new, serious adverse drug effects."[3]

How do you decide whether a case is worth reporting? Case reports involving patients should illustrate elements of patient/client management that have not yet been well described in the professional literature. Because gaps remain in the physical therapy and rehabilitation literature, a well-reasoned and clearly presented report of many types of patients would meet this criterion. A literature search—described in detail in **Chapter 3**—is necessary to determine whether a number of case reports or research reports already have been published on your topic. Even if the answer is "yes," you shouldn't automatically give up on your idea. The search results might tell you that your case report has a different angle that would make it something "new."

To get the most out of your literature search, you need to answer an important question before you begin: What's the focus of the case report that has been waiting, half-formed, in the back of your mind?

Ask yourself the most important question

Keep It Focused!

A case report involving a patient or a group of patients (no more than 10) should address all of the essential elements of patient/client management (examination, evaluation, diagnosis, prognosis, and intervention) and outcomes—but the case report may focus on one or more of them.[4] The essential elements of patient/client management provided by physical therapists are defined by the *Guide to Physical Therapist Practice*[5] (See **Chapter 6** for more).

Keeping the elements of patient/client management in mind, how might you focus your case report? Because so many different aspects of physical therapy can be described in a case report, *PTJ* decided that a "one-size-fits-all" approach is insufficient and established 7 focus-based case report formats:

- Diagnosis/Prognosis
- Intervention
- Application of Theory to Practice
- Administrative/Educational Process
- Clinical Measurement Procedures
- Risk Management
- "Full," Traditional Case Report

Regardless of the journal you're considering for your case report, a focused approach might be valuable. Below we describe these focuses and provide some—but only some— illustrative examples of the approaches you could take.

Diagnosis/Prognosis

Focus on the process and logic associated with differential diagnosis (ie, clinical decision making), unusual or difficult diagnostic or prognostic events, or missed diagnoses. Detail should be concentrated in the patient history and physical examination and in the conclusion or decisions made based on the examination. Your case report should challenge readers to deduce the diagnosis and to determine how the diagnosis relates to the care of the patient. Interventions and outcomes may be included but would not be as detailed. You might...

- **Select a patient whose diagnosis was difficult to make.** Your report would highlight your decision-making processes related to the examination, evaluation, and diagnosis. The rich description of this process could then be followed by a briefer, but replicable, description of the intervention (if any) and the outcomes. Consider the case report about an underlying— and undetected—hangman's fracture in a patient with neck pain referred for physical therapy.[6] The 61-year-old man had a sudden onset of neck pain 8 weeks after a motor vehicle accident, but conventional cervical spine radiographs taken on the day of the accident did not show any abnormalities. Based on initial examination findings, the physical therapist wanted to rule out the possibility of an undetected fracture and ordered further conventional radiographs, which were consistent with a hangman's fracture. This case report had a clear message: "In patients with neck pain caused by trauma, physical therapists should be alert for the presence of cervical spine fractures. Even if the initial radiographs are negative for a

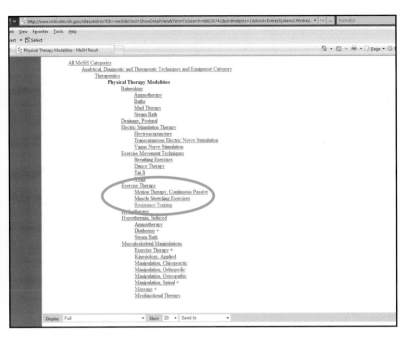

FIGURE 6B. Click on "physical therapy modalities" and find that the definition of "physical therapy modalities" includes exercise.

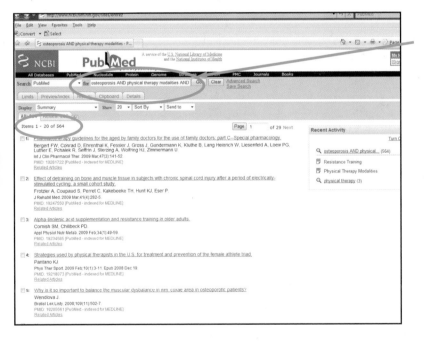

FIGURE 7. In the PubMed query box, enter **osteoporosis AND physical therapy modalities**, and click on the Go button. PubMed searches for these terms in the title, abstract, and MeSH categories of each citation—and produces more than 500 matches.

Step 2: **Begin your search.** You go to the PubMed search screen. In the query box, you type **osteoporosis AND physical therapy modalities**, and click on the Go button (**Figure 7**). PubMed searches for these terms in the title, abstract, and MeSH categories of each citation—and produces more than 500 matches. This means that your search was too wide.

FIGURE 8. In the PubMed query box, enter **osteoporosis AND physical therapy modalities AND weight-bearing exercise**, and click on the Go button. PubMed searches for these terms in the title, abstract, and MeSH categories of each citation— and produces a much more manageable total of 51 matches.

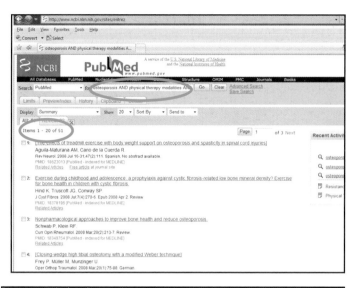

FIGURE 9. Click the Limits tab to set limits on your search. Select English and check the "Abstracts" box. After clicking the Go button, you see that PubMed limits the search based on your criteria.

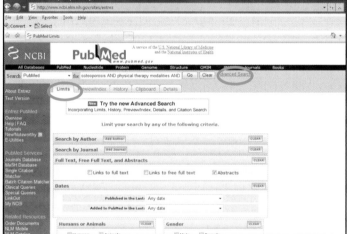

Step 3: Narrow your search. To search for case reports that are similar to your case, you need to conduct a winnowing process. Because you are particularly interested in weight-bearing exercise for your patient, you type **osteoporosis AND physical therapy modalities AND weight-bearing exercise** in the query box. This yields 51 articles—a much more manageable number (**Figure 8**).

In scanning the article titles, you notice that these search results include research on children. To further narrow your search, PubMed offers a number of different options. First, you click on the Limits tab to set limits on your search: fields within the citation (eg, title, journal, MeSH heading), publication type (eg, clinical trial, case report, review, randomized clinical trial, meta-analysis), language, age group, human or animal study, gender, citations with abstract (a check box), and publication date (**Figure 9**). You select "English" and check the "Abstracts" box. After you click on the Go button, PubMed limits the search based on your criteria.

Your search produces about 41 citations. To further refine your search, you click the Limits tab again, click on "Case Reports" under "Type of Article," then click Go. This narrows the yield to 4 citations (**Figure 10**).

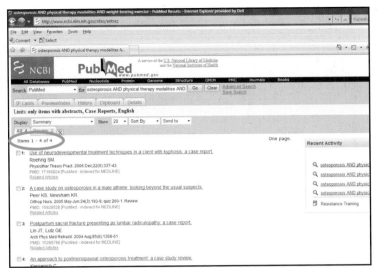

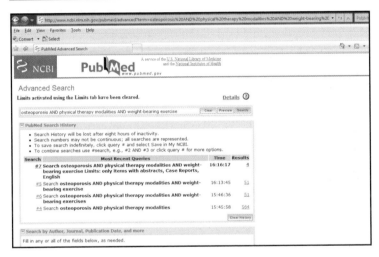

FIGURE 10. To further refine your search, click the Limits tab again, click on "Case Reports" under "Type of Article," then click Go. This narrows the yield to 4 citations.

FIGURE 11. PubMed offers an advanced search option that allows users to incorporate limits, search history, citation search, and more in one search.

You can further limit your search to sex or certain patient populations (in this case, you select "Female" and "Aged: 65+ years"). This yields 2 citations.

To search for articles written by a particular author, you can clear the query box and type in the author's last name followed by first and middle initial, and PubMed then pulls up every article in the database written by that author. (Be aware that PubMed might list the same author using 1 or 2 initials, depending on the publication. In addition, other authors with the same last name and initials will be included in the results.) You can find out if a particular journal is listed in MEDLINE by clicking the Journals Database link under "PubMed Services" (Figure 6A).

PubMed offers an advanced search option that allows users to incorporate limits, search history, citation search, and more in one seamless search (Figure 11). You can access it directly at *http://www.ncbi.nlm.nih.gov/pubmed/advanced* or from any PubMed search page.

FIGURE 12. You also can search PubMed/MEDLINE using PICO (Patient/Problem, Intervention, Compare, Outcome).

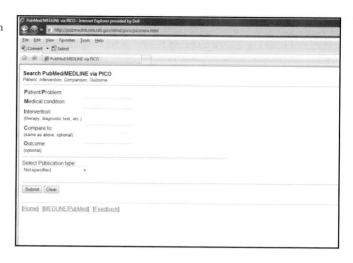

Other search options:

■ PubMed's Clinical Queries feature allows specialized PubMed searches for clinician via these links: search by clinical study category, searches for systematic reviews only, and medical genetics searches. The Limits options noted above can also be used for Clinical Query searches.

■ You can search PubMed/MEDLINE using PICO (Patient/Problem, Intervention, Compare, Outcome) (Figure 12). Go to *http://pubmedhh.nlm.nih.gov/nlmd/pico/piconew.html.*

■ You can search directly from the MeSH database when you're in PubMed. In most cases, this will *immediately* narrow your search—perhaps more than you want, so this is where your judgment will be required. Consider how it works using the terms for the basic PubMed search we just conducted. In the MeSH database, enter the term **physical therapy** in the query box, click Go, and then click in the box next to the term "physical therapy modalities." Pull down the "Send to" menu, and click "Search Box with AND." This will automatically add your terms to the search box. Next, clear the query, and enter **osteoporosis**, click the box next to the term, pull down the "Send to" menu, click "Search Box with AND," and click on the Search PubMed button. This yields under 500 citations, compared with the more than 500 matches in the basic search. Because you want to narrow your search further and are interested in weight-bearing exercise specifically, you hit the back button, clear the query, and enter **physical therapy modalities.** Scroll down the subject term tree, and click on the "Resistance training" link under "Exercise therapy." Click in the box next to "Resistance training," pull down the "Send to" menu again to add this term to your search, and click "Search Box with AND." This search yields 5 citations, compared with te 51 citations obtained when **osteoporosis AND physical therapy modalities AND weight-bearing exercise** were used in the basic search. When the same limits used in the basic search are applied to this set of search results, the yield is 0.

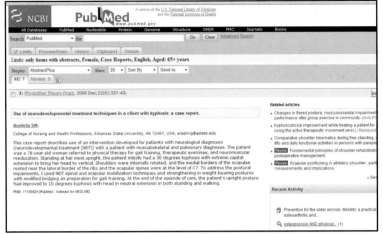

FIGURE 13. To view the abstract for a citation, click on the article title. When you find a particularly relevant article, click the Related Articles link to find similar articles. Many citations now link directly to the journal in which the article was published.

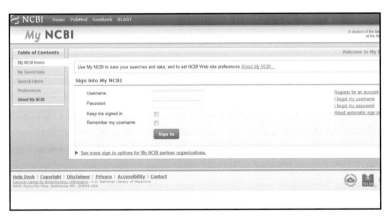

FIGURE 14. As you review the abstracts, select those articles that you believe are most pertinent to your case report. PubMed gives you the option of saving your entire search in MyNCBI.

The PubMed screens in this chapter appear courtesy of the National Library of Medicine. Remember that screens may look somewhat different depending on the online service or browser that is being used.

Step 4: Select the articles you need. Now that your search has been narrowed, you review the citations from the list produced by PubMed. The default setting for the list is "Summary," which provides the author name, title, and bibliographic information for each citation. For each abstract, the title is shown as a link. To view the abstract for a citation, click on the article title. When you find a particularly relevant article, click the Related Articles link to find similar articles (Figure 13). Many citations now link directly to the journal in which the article was published.

As you review the abstracts, select those articles that you believe are most pertinent to your case report. PubMed gives you the option of saving your entire search (Figure 14), using a free service called "My NCBI" (National Center for Biotechnology Information). This is helpful when you want to do more than one search per session. Free, one-time registration and login are required.

Obtaining Articles

There are a number of ways to obtain full text of the articles that you want:

- Many if not most PubMed citations link directly to the Web site of the journal that published the article. Although journal Web sites may require a subscription or membership in a professional association to access full text, you usually will have the option of obtaining access to a particular article through pay-per-view. You may be able to access older material without charge, depending on the journal's "embargo" policy: many journals make all articles free 12 months after publication. In addition, medical libraries and perhaps some public libraries may have subscriptions to journal Web sites either individually or as a bundled subscription, in which case you could log on to the journal Web site from the library.

- Your library may store textbooks in the stacks; journals in a special periodicals room, in the stacks, or on microfiche or microfilm; and government documents grouped together in a special location. Consult the library's online catalog to find the call number of a particular item. If you have problems locating an item, a librarian can help.

- If the library does not have the item you need, you can request an interlibrary loan. The librarian can locate the journal or book using the citation you provide. Other libraries (in the same city or in a different state or region) will lend you a book or send you a copy of the article. The interlibrary loan may require a fee to cover the costs of copying and postage. Again, check with your library for rates and fees that may apply.

- You can visit PubMed Central (*http://www.pubmedcentral.nih.gov*), which provides open access to the full text of articles that report on research funded by the National Institutes of Health and other funders.

- You can order the full text of articles through the National Library of Medicine's Loansome Doc service. If the library where you conducted your search does not offer Loansome Doc, you can contact a participating library in the National Network of Libraries of Medicine (NN/LM) to set up an account. For a list of list of libraries that provide Loansome Doc service, call NN/LM at 800/338-7657. More information about Loansome Doc, including questions that you should ask your provider, is available online at *http://www.nlm.nih.gov/loansomedoc/loansome_home.html*. Other document delivery services include those operated by university and public libraries or by commercial document delivery services such as *http://DocDel.net*.

- If an article is fairly recent, you may be able to contact the author for a reprint. If the article was published several years ago, however, you might not be able to locate the author. You can start by checking the PubMed abstract for the primary author's email address, or simply type the title of the article into Google search. You may be surprised at the number of full-text articles you can get this way!

- Remember: Don't forget the obvious! Ask your colleagues if they have access to a particular publication.

Incorporating the Search Into Your Case Report

It's not necessary (or even desirable) to write about your actual literature search. It's far more important to spend time integrating the search results into the background and purpose of your case report.

In their case report about gait characteristics of a soldier with a traumatic hip disarticulation, Schnall and colleagues[6] talked about the types of evidence—and paucity of evidence—available related to their topic. They noted when a case report was the only available literature that contained kinematic information relevant to their case as well as the limited amount of research to assist clinicians:

> As a result of the recent conflicts in Afghanistan and Iraq, US soldiers have incurred complex injuries. Between 2002 and June 2007, 14 soldiers had sustained a hip disarticulation (HD), with 8 having unilateral amputations and 6 having multiple limb involvement.[1] Military personnel who are young, premorbidly fit, and goal oriented pose new challenges for rehabilitation professionals, as there is little to no research on this population to guide prognosis of function and gait training or to understand their prosthetic demands. The incidence of HD surgeries among patients with amputations has been reported as 0.5% to 3.0%.[2-4] Most of these surgeries are due to vascular impairment or malignancy and tend to have poor outcomes.[4,5] Of those patients who have the ability to walk, many opt for prosthesis-free crutch walking.[6] As a result of the small number of prosthetic users with this diagnosis, limited research is available to guide clinicians in their care and rehabilitation.…
>
> Unfortunately, no documentation of kinetic data has been reported in the literature, and few studies have reported kinematic and metabolic data. One case study reporting kinematic data involved a 73-year-old man with cardiopulmonary disease,[7] so the results may not generalize to a younger population.…

More about integrating the results of your literature search in **Chapter 6.**

NEXT

You've Chosen a Case—Are You Ready to Write?
You've reviewed the literature and found no case reports or research articles on your exact topic. You've even found the literature to support the importance of your topic and the credibility of your patient/client management. You're almost ready to start writing! But first, you have some important "almost-writing" tasks. You need to think about operational definitions—and the measurements that you'll use.

References

1 Kelo MJ, Riddle DL. Examination and management of a patient with tarsal coalition. *Phys Ther.* 1998;78:518-525.

2 Levels of evidence. Centre for Evidence-based Medicine. Available at http://www.cebm.net/index.aspx?0=1025. Accessed April 24, 2009.

3 Davidoff F. Masking, blinding, and peer review: the blind leading the blinded [editorial]. *Ann Intern Med.* 1998;128:66-68.

4 Rothstein JM. Peer review [editor's note]. *Phys Ther.* 1991;71:88-89.

5 *Medical and Health Care Books and Serials in Print*, vols 1 and 2. New Providence, NJ: Bowker; 2008.

6 Schnall BL, Baum BS, Andrews AM. Gait characteristics of a soldier with a traumatic hip disarticulation. *Phys Ther.* 2008;88:1568-1577.

CHAPTER 4

Defining and Measuring

Everyone *doesn't* know what you mean! Make certain that others will be able to replicate what you did.

Have you ever read patient charts and wondered what the treating therapist meant when describing the patient, an examination, or an intervention procedure? Part of the problem is that therapists often use jargon or ambiguous terms. We use these terms because we think that "everyone knows what they mean." But "everyone" doesn't know what those terms mean! Does "moderate assistance" really indicate how much you have to help the patient? When you read, "I cleared the patient's neck," do you know what procedures were used? If treatment is said to include "balance training," will you be able to replicate it? Exactly what is "conventional physical therapy"? How would another clinician recognize and replicate a "spongy end feel" or a "press up"?

Operationalize!

Because a case report is the purest description of how we practice, operational definitions are an essential ingredient. No matter what topic the case report covers, the interactions between the author and the patient (or other entity) must be "operationalized." Operational definitions traditionally have been viewed as descriptions of what to look for, what to do, and how to obtain a measurement. When we operationally define something, we describe all of the steps involved in completing a task.

Operational definitions allow us to replicate and interpret the measurements obtained by others—and ourselves. For example, if we all take a measurement in the same way—that is, if we all follow the same operational definition—we get the same result (or almost the same result). In the absence of operational definitions, each of us may use a different set of rules to take a measurement, greatly increasing the chances for error. The position of the patient, for example, can make a difference in a range-of-motion measurement. Time of day, type of floor surface, type of footwear, and medication all are factors that can affect the distance that a patient walks or the amount of assistance that a patient needs to dress. Clear descriptions of these and any other relevant conditions reduce the chances of measurement error.

For the purpose of case reports, the classic term "operational definition" should be broadened to apply not only to measurements but to patient histories, interventions, and outcomes. The reader should be able to:

- Identify patients who have characteristics similar to those of the patient(s) in the case report.
- Replicate the medical history and examination procedures.
- Replicate the intervention.
- Assess the outcome of the intervention in a similar way.
- Understand the author's clinical reasoning process.

Tips on providing operational definitions will be given throughout this manual. This chapter focuses on measurement reliability and validity—the "two-headed monster" that is closely related to operational definitions. Remember that you don't need to address measurement properties for *all* measurements related to your case—only the key measurements.

What Constitutes a Measurement?

To describe patient examinations and outcomes—and sometimes interventions—clinicians have to take measurements. APTA's *Standards for Tests and Measurements in Physical Therapy Practice*[1(p12)] defines *measurement* as "the numeral assigned to an object, event, or person or the class (category) to which an object, event, or person is assigned according to rules." This definition implies that any time a therapist assesses something based on a set of rules or steps, the therapist has taken a measurement.

What constitutes a measurement can be very subtle. When you determine the extent of assistance that a patient requires to dress, you are taking a measurement. When you assess the magnitude of a patient's report of pain, you are taking a measurement. When you observe and subsequently describe a patient's gait pattern, you are taking a measurement. In a case report, these and all other types of measurements must meet at least minimal requirements of reliability and validity. Why? In case reports, measurements are taken for only one patient or a few patients at a time, unlike studies with large numbers of subjects. It is especially important that the therapist (and the reader) have confidence that the measurements accurately reflect the patient's condition.

The two-headed monster of reliability and validity strikes fear into almost every clinician's heart—but the reality is that the clinician deals with that monster every day.

What Is Your Purpose for Measurement?

To accurately reflect a patient's condition, tests and measures must be selected with the purpose of the measurement in mind. Is the purpose to diagnosis a condition? Is the purpose to measure change with intervention, or change over time? Or is the purpose to predict something about the future?

Kirshner and Guyatt[2] described 3 purposes for clinical measurement: discrimination, prediction, and evaluation. Discriminative measurements identify patients with or without a particular characteristic or with varying degrees of a characteristic, such as decreased strength or range of motion, impaired balance, anterior cruciate ligament (ACL) rupture, or delayed gross motor skills. Good discriminative tools are useful for identifying whether a patient has a particular problem, and they contribute useful information for the process of diagnosis.

Evaluative measurements are used to assess change over time or as a result of intervention.[2] Good evaluative measurements are responsive to change that occurs, whether in body structures and functions, activity, or participation. Good discriminative measurements are not necessarily good evaluative measurements. Many discriminative measurements either cannot measure change that occurs (see **Chapter 5**) or do not measure things that are important to the patient. Patients usually care more about their ability to function in their daily lives than about their muscle performance or range of motion.

Predictive measurements are used to identify which patients have or are likely to have a particular condition or status in the future.[2] For this reason, predictive measures are particularly useful when attempting to determine a patient's prognosis. The Test of Infant Motor Performance,[3] for example, predicts which infants at risk for abnormal motor development will later be diagnosed with conditions such as cerebral palsy; and researchers have used the Lower-Extremity Functional Scale (LEFS) and the Six-Minute Walk Test (6MWT) to predict the expected rate of improvement and total improvement in people following total knee arthroplasty.[4]

Research is necessary to know if and how well measurements serve their purposes (validity, sensitivity, specificity, and other measurement properties are discussed later in this chapter). Case report authors are not expected to *do* this research, but they are expected to know whether the research exists and to use that information when deciding which tests and measures are most appropriate for their patients and when interpreting the measurements.

No matter what the purpose of the measurement, accurate reflection of the patient's condition also requires measurements to be accurate—this is where reliability comes in.

> You don't need to *do* the research, but you do need to *know* the research

Reliability: Accounting for Error

The reliability of the measurement indicates how much error exists in the measurement. All measurements have at least a little error, but too much error makes a measurement meaningless. Where does error come from? A variety of sources:

■ **Examiner error.** Examiners contribute error to a measurement when they do not follow the operational definition of the examination procedure. When a therapist measures the range of motion at a joint but does not align the goniometer properly, for example, error occurs. Error also occurs when a therapist does not follow the instructions for administering a standardized test.

■ **Instrument error.** How many times have you measured range of motion with a goniometer that had a loose screw that prevented you from reading the angle properly? Instruments aren't limited to devices or machines; they also can be the written instructions (operational definitions again) that must be used to obtain a measurement, such as a set of rules to classify a patient's movement pattern. When the set of rules is not understandable (ie, operational), it can be considered to be faulty and may add error to the measurement.

■ **Patient error.** The patient as a source of error in clinical practice may be a difficult concept to understand. If you assess the force production of a patient's biceps 3 hours after surgery and compare that measurement with one taken the next day, the 2 measurements will be different. The difference, however, doesn't represent true change in the force-producing capacity of the biceps muscle. Changes in force-production capability can take weeks to occur. The difference may relate to the fact that the patient still was experiencing effects from the anesthesia during the first test. When patient-related factors such as this one influence a measurement, error results.

Measurement error can be minimized only when therapists do everything they can do to eliminate the possible sources of error. The higher the reliability for a single measurement—that is, the more assured we can be that examiner, instrument, or patient errors are minimal—the more likely the measurement is to represent the true status of the patient. High reliability is particularly important when repeated measurements are taken over time to assess change in a patient's status. Small changes in highly reliable measurements are likely to indicate a real change in the patient's condition, whereas small changes in lower-reliability measurements are likely to reflect error.

What Is Acceptable Reliability?

The word "acceptable" requires clarification. Reliability coefficients often are used to indicate the degree of agreement between measurements. Coefficients can be calculated using a variety of statistics, but the resulting numbers generally are interpreted in the same way. These numbers can represent agreement between measurements taken by different testers (*intertester reliability*) or by the same tester (*intratester reliability*). A reliability coefficient is a number between 0 and 1.0, with 0 indicating no agreement and 1.0 indicating perfect agreement. Numbers that are closer to 1.0, such as .95, indicate better agreement than do numbers that are lower, such as .65. Portney and Watkins[5] recommended a general guideline for interpreting coefficients, but they cautioned that the purpose of the measurement must be considered and that the coefficients are only a starting point for judging acceptable standards for a measurement:

0 to .50 = poor reliability
.50 to .75 = moderate reliability
75 to 1.0 = good reliability

What is an acceptable level of agreement for a case report? Portney and Watkins[5] suggested that most clinical measurements should have a reliability of at least .90. Acceptable reliability depends on how precisely the variable can be measured and how the measurement will be interpreted and used. Remember that these estimates are only guidelines. For instance, if the reliability coefficient for a measure is .95, you can be reasonably confident that relatively small changes represent real change. If the coefficient is .70, however, relatively large changes would have to occur to indicate real change. (See **Chapter 5** for more about measuring change.)

How Can You Show That Your Measurements Are Reliable?

Strategy 1: Reference Previously Published Reliability Studies

This may be the most common and most sound way of providing evidence for acceptable reliability of measurements in a case report. Reliability studies usually are designed with large numbers of patients and therapists, which enhances the generalizability of the findings. Therapists who use tests and measures that have acceptable levels of reliability estimated through research can be reasonably certain that their measurements are reliable, assuming that they followed the operational definitions or standardized procedures for the measurement. If you cite a previously published study to support the reliability of the measurements you obtained, make certain you explain how you followed the operational definitions or standardized procedures. It is also important to ensure that the measurements you report were taken by therapists who have been trained similarly to those who took the measurements in the published reliability study. *The pertinent characteristics of the patient or patients in the case report should be similar to those of the subjects in the reliability study.*

> Explain how you followed the procedure described in the literature

Cernak et al[6] used the transfer and locomotion subscales of the Pediatric Functional Independence Measure (WeeFIM) to measure mobility in a child with ataxia with whom they used a body-weight–supported treadmill training. Here is how they described the reliability of these measurements[6(pp90-91)]:

> Interrater reliability is high (intraclass correlation coefficient [ICC]=.90–.99), as is test-retest reliability (ICC=.98–.99).[22] Ottenbacher et al[22] also demonstrated that the ICC was the highest (.99) for the transfers and locomotion subscales that we used with our patient.

By indicating the statistic used to estimate reliability (ICC), the authors let readers know that, unlike correlation coefficients such as Pearson r, the coefficient reflects both degree of correspondence and agreement among ratings.[5] By reporting the ICC values, they informed readers about the strength of the reliability, which is more useful than simply saying reliability was "high." Reliability considered high for one purpose might not be considered high for another purpose. The authors also informed readers by reporting the types of reliability (interrater and test-retest) and did not simply report "reliability." Because the authors used only 2 subscales of the Wee-FIM, reporting the reliability of those subscales also was important. Reliability of the entire measure might not be the same as the reliability of individual subscale measurements.

In a similar way, Prosser[7] reported the reliability of measurements that she used in her case report of a child with incomplete spinal cord injury. When describing the child's scores on the American Spinal Injury Association (ASIA) Impairment Scale, she wrote:

> The patient's initial ASIA sensory score was 26/224 (initial pinprick score=12/112, initial light touch score=14/112), including impaired light touch in the right S3 and S4–5

dermatomes.... The reliability of ASIA scores in children 6 to 11 years of age have been reported.[22] Intraclass correlation coefficients (ICC) with 95% confidence intervals were .711 (.226–.892) for total motor score, .952 (.867–.983) for pinprick score, and .952 (.867–.983) for light touch score.[22]

(A side note: *PTJ* now asks authors to report ICC to 2 decimals, not 3, as we just don't have that much precision.)

Because the child in the case report was 5 years old and the reliability study included children aged 6 to 11 years, the author could have added a comment about why she thought the results of the study could be generalized to her patient. The type of reliability the study estimated also would have been informative.

Vaughn and Nitsch[8] used the literature to support the reliability of their measurements of a patient's knee when they wrote:

Gogia et al[44] have reported intraclass correlation coefficients of .98 for intertester reliability ... for goniometric measurement of the knee. End-feels were assessed at the end of the range of motion and were classified as hard, firm, or soft.[45] The reliability of end-feel measurements has not been demonstrated.

Note that the authors acknowledged that reliability data did not exist for classification of end-feels. When reliability data do not exist, authors should consider the possibility of error when explaining the contribution that the measurements made to decision making.

Crow et al[9] also referenced the literature to support the reliability of an outcome measure, the Harris Hip Score (HHS). The following excerpt exemplifies using the literature to support not only the reliability of a measure, but the application of a minimal clinically important difference (see **Chapter 5**):

Kirmit et al[13] reported that the HHS (Harris Hip Score) has excellent interobserver reliability (kappa=.91). Hoeksma et al[14] reported a minimal clinically important difference of 4 points for the HHS.... Total disability, as measured by the HHS, demonstrated a 13-point improvement (from 83 points at baseline to 96 points at discharge) and was clinically significant (Tab. 2).

Many case reports include measurements taken with instruments that, no matter how high tech, cannot be assumed to provide reliable measurements. Hastings et al[10] used quantitative computed topography (QCT) to measure bone mineral density (BMD) of their patient's foot. They supported the reliability and validity of the measurements this way:

Prior research has established evidence of the validity of the QCT (quantitative computed tomography) as a technique for the measurement of foot BMD.[22] Absolute measurement error was computed as the bias (mean) and root-mean-square standard deviation of the difference in BMD between repeated scans for the tarsals and metatarsals. The bias was small (−3.1 to 0.5), and reliability (root-mean-square standard deviation) was 3.1 mg/cm3.[22]

You can find many published reliability studies through a literature search. **Chapter 3** gives tips for searching the literature to find these and other types of research.

Strategy 2: Conduct a Mini-Reliability Study

When measurements have not been adequately studied previously for reliability, or when you want to make sure your own measurements are reliable, you have the option of doing a mini-reliability study as part of the case report. When Jones et al[11] described the use of power mobility for a young child with spinal muscular atrophy, for example, they reported the published reliability of the Battelle Developmental Inventory (BDI) and the PEDI, and they also reported the reliability of their own measurements:

> The BDI test manual reports intraclass correlation coefficients (ICC) ranging between .90 and .99 for test-retest reliability and interrater reliability of the BDI total scores in a combined normative and clinical sample of 183 children. Using the Cohen Kappa, we calculated the interrater reliability of the BDI total scores … and coefficients ranged between .92 and .98.
>
> The PEDI manual reports good internal consistency, with coefficients ranging between .95 and .99 for all 6 scales using Cronbach coefficient alpha. The test developers used the ICC to calculate inter-interviewer reliability, and coefficients ranged from .96 to .99 on all scales in a normative sample of 30 children and from .84 to 1.00 in a clinical sample of 12 children. Using the Cohen Kappa, we calculated the inter-interviewer reliability of the PEDI total scores and the functional skills and caregiver assistance scales … and achieved coefficients between .92 and 1.00.

Bad measurement humor: 1,000,000 aches = 1 megahurtz

Reliability estimates from mini-reliability studies are more limited than those from larger reliability studies, and the number of subjects in a mini-reliability study is usually too small to generalize to other settings. Whenever possible, therefore, larger reliability studies still should be referenced.

A mini-reliability study is not required, but it isn't difficult to do. It just takes some time to set up the study and to obtain and analyze the repeated measurements. The purpose of the mini-reliability study is to determine the consistency of measurements taken more than once by the same clinician (intratester reliability) or taken by 2 or more clinicians (intertester reliability).

When 2 sets of measurements are taken by one tester, it is important to "mask" the results from the tester if remembering the measurement could cause bias. When measuring range of motion, for example, tape can be placed over the numbers on the side of the goniometer visible to the tester, and another clinician can read and record the results. Some measurements are difficult or impossible to mask and easy to remember. In these cases, the better course of action might be to determine intertester reliability. Intertester reliability also should be determined when more than one clinician is taking measurements throughout a patient's episode of care.

The type of statistical analysis to use depends on the type of data and other factors that are too numerous to explain in this manual. The book by Portney and Watkins[5] is one good source of information about reliability studies and should be useful for clinicians who have minimal background in research design and statistics. Other research and statistics texts also can give good advice. If you don't feel up to dealing with a mini-reliability study on your own, don't hesitate to ask for help from local university faculty or other colleagues with knowledge in this area.

Strategy 3: Make a Presumptive Argument

With this strategy, the author essentially develops a theoretical argument that supports the notion that the measurement adequately represents the variable of interest and has an acceptable level of reliability. This method should be the method of last resort, however, and should be used only when published reliability studies do not exist and you choose not to do a mini-reliability study (eg, when reporting a case retrospectively).

An acceptable presumptive argument often is simply an explanation of what you do in the clinic to ensure that measurement error is minimized. Depending on the type of measurement and your knowledge of likely sources of measurement error, you could explain how you ensured that the patient was positioned in the same way each time, was always measured at the same time of day, or was measured by the same therapist each time (intratester reliability is usually higher than intertester reliability), using written operational definitions of the measurement procedure. Most presumptive arguments simply describe good clinical measurement practices.

Kaufman and Schilling[12] used some of these explanations when they made a presumptive argument for the reliability of their handheld dynamometer measurements of a child with developmental coordination disorder:

> Originally, manual muscle testing was attempted, but it was not continued due to Andy's inability to follow instructions, as demonstrated by inconsistency and repetitive muscle substitution. Muscle testing then was successfully performed using a handheld dynamometer (HHD) to establish baseline and posttraining strength measurements as well as data for the strength training protocol. Andy responded better to directions regarding movement using a dynamometer, and he appeared to have a decreased level of frustration and increased consistency in his performance. Measurements were taken the same time of day during his scheduled physical therapy sessions, and he was given the same rest periods between trials. Three HHD measurements obtained for each muscle tested were found to be similar and based on professional judgment were concluded to be more precise and reliable for this child.

This presumptive argument first described the child's behavior during manual muscle testing and the improvement that the authors saw when using the handheld dynamometer. The authors then explained how they attempted to control for the child as a source of error by taking the measurements at the same time of day and letting him rest between trials. Finally, they measured each muscle 3 times and the 3 measurements were similar, which argues for the consistency of the measurements.

If a strong case can be made for the reliability of the measurements, the validity of the measurements is the next issue to be address. It's important to remember that measurements can be reliable even if they are not valid, but they cannot be valid if they are not reliable. Validity of measurements in a case report, like reliability of measurements, usually can be handled adequately by descriptions of sound practice and clinical reasoning.

Validity: Using Measurement in Clinical Decisions

The validity of a measurement can be an elusive concept to understand. *Standards for Tests and Measurements in Physical Therapy Practice*[1(p15)] defines validity as the "degree to which a useful (meaningful) interpretation can be inferred from a measurement." The concept of validity relates to what the measurement is used for and how it is used in making decisions. There are 2 broad types of validity: criterion-based and theory-based (Table 2). Sensitivity, specificity, and likelihood ratios are other validity-related properties of tests and measures used for diagnosis.

Criterion-based Forms of Validity

This type of validity relates how well a measurement reflects what it is designed to reflect. Does a test purported to measure balance, for example, produce measurements that reflect the construct of balance, or do the measurements really reflect a patient's ability to understand instructions? Does a test developed to identify newborn infants who will later be diagnosed as having cerebral palsy succeed in this prediction? Does performance on a test in the clinic relate to a patient's performance at home? Table 2 includes definitions of some types of criterion-based validity (concurrent validity, predictive validity, and prescriptive validity). These and other forms of criterion-based validity are discussed thoroughly in the *Primer on Measurement*[13] and in other reference works.

The criterion-based forms of validity are studied in research by correlating measurements obtained using the tool of interest with measurements obtained using an already validated tool, or the *criterion measure* or "gold standard." The validity of the tool of interest is assessed by determining how well its measurements correlate with those of the criterion measure. The correlation coefficients are interpreted in the same way that reliability coefficients are interpreted, with correlations closer to 1.0 indicating a stronger relationship between the measurements of interest and the criterion measurements. If, for example, children's scores on a new quick test of motor development had a correlation coefficient of .90 with an established test of motor development, the quick test would have strong concurrent validity with the criterion test and might be used in place of it. On the other hand, if the correlation between the height of basketball players' vertical jump on one foot and the number of rebounds during the season was .25, vertical jump height would have poor predictive validity for number of rebounds.

> The concept of validity may seem elusive, but all it really means is how a measurement is used in making clinical decisions.

Research on the criterion-related validity is available for an increasing number of tests and measures, as indicated by the following examples. In their case report of a rehabilitation program for patients with chronic heart failure (CHF), Nilsson and colleagues[14] described the criterion-based validity of the 6MWT:

> The 6MWT has been shown to be valid for walking capacity and physical activity in patients with CHF[28] and closely mimics the daily submaximal energy expenditure required for functional activities.[28] The distance covered during the 6MWT has been shown to be closely related to exercise capacity indexes of bicycle work rate, stair-climbing time, and peak oxygen consumption.[29]

TABLE 2. Definitions and Examples of Types of Validity[a]

Criterion-Based Forms of Validity

Concurrent validity: Inferred interpretations are justified by comparing a measurement with supporting evidence that was obtained at approximately the same time that the measurement being validated was obtained. If measurements using a simple and inexpensive test to detect balance problems could be shown to be related to measurements using sophisticated and expensive equipment, the simple test then could be used in place of and interpreted in the same way as the expensive test, because the tests have good concurrent validity.

Predictive validity: Inferred interpretations are justified by comparing a measurement with supporting evidence obtained at a later point in time. That is, predictive validity involves the justification of the use of a measurement to say something about future events or conditions. We frequently base our decisions on tests that we assume predict the future, but little evidence exists to support the predictive validity of many of these tests. Do preseason screenings of football players, motor assessments of infants, and preemployment tests actually predict later performance or injury?

Prescriptive validity: Inferred interpretation of a measurement is the determination of the form of intervention that a person is to receive. That is, prescriptive validity is justified based on the successful outcome of the chosen intervention. If results of a test to determine the cause of patients' low back pain led to a specific intervention that resulted in patients' return to work, the test would have prescriptive validity.

Theoretical Forms of Validity

Construct validity: The conceptual (theoretical) basis for using a measurement to make an inferred interpretation. Knowledge of reflexes, the nervous system, and neuropathology could provide a theoretical basis for the development of both a testing procedure (eg, the reflex hammer) and a measurement (eg, the reflex response). This knowledge, a theoretical underpinning, is the construct on which the test and measurement are developed.

Content validity: A theoretical form of validity that deals with the extent to which a measurement is judged to reflect the meaningful elements of a construct and not any extraneous elements. Content validity is closely related to construct validity. The "construct" of balance could be defined with knowledge of structures and mechanisms believed to contribute to balance. The content validity of a test to measure balance would then be judged by its ability to measure the relevant structures and mechanisms, and not extra elements that don't relate to balance or conflicting elements, such as a patient's ability to follow instructions.

[a] Information adapted with permission of the American Physical Therapy Association from Rothstein JM, Echternach JL. Primer on Measurement: An Introductory Guide to Measurement Issues. *Alexandria, VA: American Physical Therapy Association; 1993.*

Because criterion-related validity might not be the same for all patient groups, reporting validity research conducted with patients with CHF was important. If research with patients with CHF had not been available, the authors might have been able to make a presumptive argument for the generalizability of research with other patient groups. If the authors had given correlation coefficients for the association of the 6MWT with the other measures, that information would have been useful for readers.

Fragala-Pinkham[15] and colleagues reported the criterion-based validity of many of the measures that they used in their case report of a fitness program for children with disabilities. This is what they wrote about the energy expenditure index:

> Walking efficiency was measured using the energy expenditure index (EEI).[27,28] ... The EEI ... has been validated.[28-31] For children with and without cerebral palsy, concurrent validity of EEI data and oxygen uptake was demonstrated by Rose et al[29] when no significant differences were found between the 2 measures at a variety of walking speeds. Most recently, Norman et al[31] demonstrated concurrent validity of the oxygen consumption index and the EEI for 10 children with cerebral palsy ($r=.61$). Kramer and MacPhail[32] administered the EEI at both comfortable and fast speeds to 17 adolescents with mild cerebral palsy 2 times at each of 2 sessions held 1 week apart and reported test-retest reliability values (r) ranging from .81 to .94.

Although reports of validity studies are becoming increasingly available in the literature, they are not available for all tests and measures that clinicians use. If a study is not available to support the validity of a measurement, case report authors might be able to make a theoretical argument for usefulness.

Theory-based Forms of Validity

The 2 theoretical forms of validity are *construct validity* and *content validity* (Table 2). Like criterion-based forms of validity, construct validity and content validity are formally assessed by research. Construct validation is an ongoing process, and evidence of construct validity can be assessed using a variety of methods.[5] One of these is the *known groups method*, which determines whether a test can discriminate between those known to have a condition and those known to not have the condition. Another method is to correlate scores on a test with scores on other tests intended to measure the same construct (convergent validity) or different construct (discriminant validity).[5] Research methods texts, such as the book by Portney and Watkins,[5] explain this and other methods that case report authors might find during a search for literature on the validity of their measures. Piva and colleagues[16] discussed research on convergent validity of their measures in a case report of exercise and neuromuscular electrical stimulation for patients with rheumatoid arthritis. This is what they said about the convergent validity of the LEFS:

> The LEFS[36] is a 20-item patient self-report survey that is intended for use in patients with pathologies affecting lower-extremity function. This scale queries patients on their ability to perform general activities of daily living, general recreational activities, specific daily physical tasks, and specific recreational or occupational related tasks. ... The correlation (r) between

the LEFS and the physical function subscale of the 36-Item Short-Form Health Survey (SF-36) was .80.[36,37]

In their case report, Culp and Romani[17] described convergent validity for the Disabilities of the Arm, Shoulder, and Hand (DASH) questionnaire. Notice that the SF-36 was used to correlate with both the LEFS (above) and the DASH. The negative correlation between the DASH and the SF-36 indicates that a higher score on one test was associated with a lower score on the other test:

> The patient completed the Disabilities of the Arm, Shoulder and Hand (DASH) questionnaire and Sports/Music or Work Module as a self-report measure of function. The DASH has been validated against the Medical Outcomes Study 36-Item Short-Form Health Survey (SF-36) (–.36 to –.62)[33] and other joint-specific measures, including the Brigham (carpal tunnel) questionnaire and the Shoulder Pain and Disability Index (SPADI) (r>.69).[34]

Content validity is the other theory-based form of validity. A measurement tool has content validity if it covers the universe of the construct it purports to measure and does not measure anything else.[5] A test of balance, for example, should have items that measure balance—not a patient's ability to follow instructions. Researchers usually study content validity by asking a panel of experts to review a tool, and then modify it based on the experts' input.

Presumptive Arguments for Why a Measurement Has Construct Validity

Cited research provides the strongest argument for theoretical forms of validity of a measure. When research is not available, a presumptive argument can be made, just as a presumptive argument can be made for the reliability of measurements. Anderson and Tichenor,[18] for example, described the theoretical bases to support the construct validity for upper-limb tension tests, a series of tests used to determine if the cervical nerve roots and peripheral nerves are contributing to the patient's complaints. The authors then operationally defined the tests they used to collect data on a patient with a diagnosis of de Quervain tenosynovitis. The operational definitions gave support for the validity of the tests, which were logically related to the theoretical basis of the construct being tested.

In the introduction of their case report, McClure and Flowers[19] discussed what they perceived to be flaws in the theoretical bases for measurements of accessory motion in joints. They used their theoretical arguments to serve as the basis for recommending an alternative examination and intervention program for a patient with limited motion of the shoulder.

In a case report describing physical therapist management of a patient with West Nile virus, Miller et al[20] provided a presumptive argument for the construct validity of manual muscle testing:

> Manual muscle testing (MMT) was used to assess the force production deficit (or impairment of strength). Manual muscle tests were administered by the inpatient and outpatient therapists using the principles and scoring system described by Kendall et al.[26] Kendall et al contend that MMTs are a "necessary part of diagnostic procedures in the field of neuromuscular disorders,"[26(p39)] noting that MMTs were developed out of the care of patients

with poliovirus. The use of MMT also is supported by Sheets et al,[25] who listed MMT as the single examination tool for impairments of strength. Hall and Brody described MMT as "the most fundamental of all strength tests" in their text on therapeutic exercise.[27(p72)] Manual muscle testing also has been described as the "method of choice for assessing the strength of patients whose muscle test grades fall below fair,"[28(p5)] as was true for this patient.

The author of a case report may make a presumptive argument for both reliability and validity in the same discussion. When Watson and Schenkman[21] argued for videotaping the shoulder range of motion of the patient with paralysis of the serratus anterior muscle, they based their argument on issues related to both reliability and validity, suggesting that the videotape data were more reliable than were goniometric measurements and stating that the videotape data better reflected the variable of interest (movement of the scapula).

Validity of Diagnostic Tests: Sensitivity, Specificity, and Likelihood Ratios

Accurately diagnosing a patient requires astute clinical reasoning skills and careful analysis of data collected during the patient history and physical examination. Clinicians need to understand the diagnostic accuracy (validity) of specific tests and measures prior to incorporating them into the examination. Diagnostic accuracy often is expressed in terms of sensitivity, specificity, and likelihood ratios (LRs).[22] Clinicians usually do not calculate these properties, but they need to search the literature to find out if researchers have reported them, and, if so, to incorporate the properties into decision making.

Sensitivity (the true positive rate) refers to the ability of a test to identify patients who have a particular diagnosis.[22] A highly sensitive test is most optimal for ruling OUT a particular disorder, given a negative test result. The acronym "**SnNout**" can be used to remember that a test with high **S**ensitivity and a **N**egative result is good for ruling out the disorder.[22] In a study by Walton et al,[23] for example, the acromioclavicular (AC) joint tenderness test had a sensitivity of .96. Because the test had high sensitivity, a positive test would likely identify most of those who have AC joint pathology. A positive finding, however, might also incorrectly identify many of those who do not have an AC joint pathology as having the problem (potential high false positive rate). So, if the test is negative, we can be fairly confident that the patient does NOT have an AC joint disorder.

Specificity (the true negative rate) refers to the ability of a test to identify patients who do not have a particular problem.[22] A highly specific test is useful for ruling IN a particular disorder, given a positive test. The acronym "**SpPin**" can be used to remember that a test with high **S**pecificity and a **P**ositive result is good for ruling in the disorder.[22] In the study by Walton et al,[23] the O'Brien test had a specificity of .90. Because the test had high specificity, a negative test would likely identify most of those who do not have AC joint pathology. A negative finding might also incorrectly identify many of those who *do* have an AC joint pathology as not having the problem (potential high false negative rate). For this reason, a positive test would be good for identifying patients WITH an AC disorder.

Although sensitivity and specificity are clinically useful, LRs might be better diagnostic tools, because they help determine shifts in probability for specific diagnoses.[24] If a given test result doesn't change (increase or decrease) the probability that a patient has a specific condition, then the test might not be useful to guide clinical decision making. When examining a new patient, for example, a physical therapist estimates the probability that a patient has a particular diagnosis (pretest probability) based on either clinical experience or published literature on the prevalence of the disorder. The clinician then selects a test or series of tests that could alter the probability that a patient does or does not have the disorder in question (posttest probability). Likelihood ratios incorporate both sensitivity and specificity and can be used to provide a direct estimate of how a given test result changes the odds of either having the disorder or not.[25]

Because test results can be positive or negative, LRs for a given test have both positive (+LR) and negative forms (-LR). A +LR is calculated by dividing sensitivity by 1- specificity [sensitivity/ (1-specificity)]. To calculate the –LR 1, sensitivity is divided by specificity [(1- sensitivity)/ specificity]. Table 3 describes methods for interpreting LRs.[26]

If a test shows a positive result, the +LR is used to determine shifts in pretest to posttest probability that a patient has a particular diagnosis. The LR helps us shift our suspicion toward or away from a particular disorder or condition. Consider the following example: a patient reports pain after twisting and hyperextending a knee while playing basketball. Prior to the examination, the clinician estimates that the probability of an ACL rupture is 50% (pretest probability) based on published literature or clinical experience (perhaps 50% of previous patients with a hyperextension injury ended up having an ACL tear). The clinician then decides to use the Lachman test and finds it to be positive. According to Katz and Fingeroth,[27] the Lachman test has a +LR of 27.3, suggesting a conclusive shift in probability (posttest probability) that the patient has an ACL rupture.

TABLE 3. Interpretation of Likelihood Ratios.[26,a]

Positive Likelihood Ratio	Negative Likelihood Ratio	Interpretation
Greater than 10	Less than 0.1	Generate large and often conclusive shifts in probability
5-10	0.1-0.2	Generate moderate shifts in probability
2-5	0.2-0.5	Generate small but sometimes important shifts in probability
1-2	0.5-1	Alter probability to a small and rarely important degree

a Adapted from Fritz JM, Wainner RS. Examining diagnostic tests: an evidence-based perspective. Phys Ther. 2001;81:1546-1564.

Chapter 4: Defining and Measuring

You might be a physical therapist who sees a large number of patients with a certain condition—for instance, hand and wrist over-use injuries—and you often might have to judge whether carpal tunnel syndrome or some other problem exists. You'd likely want to identify 2 or 3 tests that have the strongest diagnostic accuracy. Or, you might provide large scale screening for an employer and be interested in the most sensitive (low –LR) tests for carpal tunnel syndrome. Or, you could be deciding whether to refer a patient to a surgeon, so you'd want to identify a very specific (high +LR) test. Two widely used tests are the Phalen test and Tinel sign. You might ask yourself, "Just how useful are these tests?" Here is a simple example to show you how a literature search to answer this question would work:

The therapist searches PubMed, using the Medical Subject Heading (MeSH) database, entering the term **carpal tunnel syndrome** and combining the results with **sensitivity and specificity** (MeSH), then clearing the search box, entering **Phalen test AND Tinel sign**, and clicking Search PubMed. (See **Chapter 3** for more about searching from the MeSH database in PubMed.) This search identifies more than 300 research articles! After checking a few of these articles, the therapist determines that the results vary so widely that the search hasn't been very useful. To get some help in interpreting the results of the studies, the therapist searches to see whether there is a meta-analysis that synthesizes the results of the studies.

To find a meta-analysis, the therapist limits the previous search to meta-analysis and also limits the search to articles in English. This search identifies only one systematic review that is relevant,[1] but the therapist notices a <u>Related Articles</u> link and finds that one of the related articles is another, more recent systematic review of clinical diagnosis of carpal tunnel syndrome.[2] The therapist decides to use this article not only because it's more recent, but because (unlike the other article) it provides a numerical synthesis of the studies, which makes the results easier to interpret. The authors had estimated the sensitivity and specificity of the tests by averaging the data across studies weighted by sample size. The overall estimate for the Phalen test was 68% sensitivity and 73% specificity. The overall estimate for the Tinel sign was 50% sensitivity and 77% specificity. Using this information, the therapist calculated likelihood ratios.

Test	Likelihood Ratios (LRs)	
	LR +	**LR –**
Phalen test	2.52	0.44
Tinel sign	2.17	0.65

Tests with likelihood ratios in these ranges would change the pretest probability to a small, although possibly important, degree.[3]

The therapist can obtain this article—through pay-per-view online or through interlibrary loan—to evaluate its quality and to see whether the authors included other tests in their analysis that might be useful.

With searching, there's always more than one strategy! If the therapist in this example had used the Clinical Queries feature of PubMed, for instance, the therapist could have chosen "Search by Clinical Study Category," selecting "Diagnosis" for category and "Broad sensitive search" for scope, and entering **carpal tunnel syndrome AND Phalen test AND Tinel sign**. This would have yielded 7 studies—a manageable number to sift through, though not necessarily review articles—along with related articles. The therapist also could have searched under "Find Systematic Reviews." Entering **carpal tunnel syndrome AND Phalen test AND Tinel sign** in the query box would not have yielded any studies, nor would entering **carpal tunnel syndrome AND Phalen test**. But entering **carpal tunnel syndrome AND Tinel sign** would have yielded 2 studies,[4,5] one of which did not come up in the previous searches but which might have been helpful.[5] Interestingly, entering **carpal tunnel syndrome AND Phalen** sign would pull up that same study. As emphasized in **Chapter 3**, manipulating your search terms is the key. You may need to be creative and explore the options.

References

1 Massy-Westropp N, Grimmer K, Bain G. A systematic review of the clinical diagnostic tests for carpal tunnel syndrome. J Hand Surg [Am]. 2000;25:120-107.

2 MacDermid JC, Wessel J. Clinical diagnosis of carpal tunnel syndrome: a systematic review. J Hand Ther. 2004;17:309-319.

3 Jaeschke R, Guyatt GH, Lijmer J. Diagnostic tests. In: Guyatt G, Drummond R, eds. Users' Guides to the Medical Literature: A Manual for Evidence-based Clinical Practice. Chicago, IL: American Medical Association; 2002:121-140.

4 D'Arcy CA, McGee S. The rational clinical examination. Does this patient have carpal tunnel syndrome? JAMA. 2000 Jun 21;283:3110-3117. Review.

5 Stolp-Smith KA, Pascoe MK, Ogburn PL Jr. Carpal tunnel syndrome in pregnancy: frequency, severity, and prognosis. Arch Phys Med Rehabil. 1998;79:1285-1287.

If a clinician finds a test to be negative, then the –LR is used to indicate a shift in the pretest probability that the patient does not have the disorder. For example, a new patient reports an insidious onset of burning pain and numbness down the right upper extremity. Prior to the examination the clinician estimates a pretest probability of cervical radiculopathy at 75%. The clinician uses the upper-limb tension test A (ULTTA), which is negative. Wainner and colleagues[28] showed that the ULTTA has a –LR of .12 for determining the probability that a patient has cervical radiculopathy. Hence, this results in a moderate shift in probability (posttest) that the patient doesn't have cervical radiculopathy.

The number of studies investigating the diagnostic utility of tests and measures used in physical therapist practice has increased recently. Case reports should include these data (sensitivity, specificity, and LRs) when describing the diagnostic process. An example can be seen in the case report by Ross and Cheeks.[29] The authors examined a patient with neck pain following a motor vehicle accident. They discuss the diagnostic utility of the Canadian Cervical Spine Rule[30] to further justify the need for ordering radiographs at the time of the physical therapist examination. The Canadian Cervical Spine Rule has sensitivity of 100%. Therefore, if the test was negative, the therapist could be confident that the patient did not have a clinically significant cervical spine fracture (SnNout) and that treatment could proceed. In this case, the test was positive and the patient was referred for further radiographs. Because the Canadian Cervical Spine Rule has low specificity (.43), a false positive finding is possible (identifying the possibility of a fracture but the radiographs being negative for a fracture). This is acceptable because we would rather send a patient for radiographs who does not have a facture than *not* send someone for radiographs who *does* have a fracture. In the Ross and Cheeks case report, the radiographs ultimately identified a hangman's fracture and prevented a potentially catastrophic outcome had the patient been treated with physical therapy.

Another example of using sensitivity and specificity to aid in clinical decision making is in a case series by Walsworth et al.[31] In an attempt to determine whether 5 patients with suspected neural involvement had cervical radiculopathy, the therapist used reflex testing, which has been shown to have specificity between .93 and .99 in patients with radiculopathy.[28, 32] If the test had been positive, they would have been able to rule in the presence of cervical radiculopathy (SpPin). Reflex testing was negative, however, so the authors began to consider other nerve pathologies. The therapists referred these 5 patients for electrophysiological evaluation, which resulted in a diagnosis of suprascapular neuropathy.

In their case report, Hall and colleagues[33] provided another example of the use of likelihood ratios. They examined 2 pregnant women with low back pain. In the examination process, the therapists used the posterior pelvic pain provocation test to determine if the patients had peripartum posterior pelvic pain. This test has been shown to have a +LR of 4.1,[34] indicating a small but sometimes important shift in probability with a positive test result.[26] With this information and other data obtained during the examination, the therapist made a provisional diagnosis of peripartum posterior pelvic pain and initiated treatment.

NEXT

Did the Patient Improve?

You've taken measurements during the examination to identify patient characteristics—such as balance skills, range of motion, or gross motor development—that contribute information for the process of diagnosis. But discriminative tests that are useful for this purpose are not necessarily useful for measuring change over time or change following intervention. An evaluative test is needed to measure change—and not all discriminative tests are good evaluative tests. Now it's time to consider some measurement concepts and properties that are important in measuring changes in your patient's status.

References

1 *Standards for Tests and Measurements in Physical Therapy Practice.* Alexandria, VA: American Physical Therapy Association; 1991.

2 Kirshner B, Guyatt B. A methodological framework for assessing health and disease. *J Chronic Dis.* 1985;38:27-36.

3 Kolobe TH, Bulanda M, Susman L. Predicting motor outcome at preschool age for infants tested at 7, 30, and 90 days after term age using the Test of Infant Motor Performance. *Phys Ther.* 2004;84:1144-1156.

4 Kennedy DM, Stratford PW, Riddle DL, et al. Assessing recovery and establishing prognosis following total knee arthroplasty. *Phys Ther.* 2008;88:22-32.

5 Portney LG, Watkins MP. *Foundations of Clinical Research: Applications to Practice.* 3rd ed. Upper Saddle River, NJ: Prentice Hall; 2009.

6 Cernak K, Stevens V, Price R, Shumway-Cook A. Locomotor training using body-weight support on a treadmill in conjunction with ongoing physical therapy in a child with severe cerebellar ataxia. *Phys Ther.* 2008;88:88-97.

7 Prosser LA. Locomotor training within an inpatient rehabilitation program after pediatric incomplete spinal cord injury. *Phys Ther.* 2007;87:1224-1232.

8 Vaughn HT, Nitsch W. Ilial anterior rotation hypermobility in a female collegiate tennis player. *Phys Ther.* 2008;88:1578-1590.

9 Crow JB, Gelfand B, Su EP. Use of joint mobilization in a patient with severely restricted hip motion following bilateral hip resurfacing arthroplasty. *Phys Ther.* 2008;88:1591-1600.

10 Hastings MK, Gelber J, Commean PK, et al. Bone mineral density of the tarsals and metatarsals with reloading. *Phys Ther.* 2008;88:766-779.

11 Jones MA, McEwen IR, Hansen L. Use of power mobility for a young child with spinal muscular atrophy. *Phys Ther.* 2003;83:253-262.

12 Kaufman LB, Schilling DL. Implementation of a strength training program for a 5-year-old child with poor body awareness and developmental coordination disorder. *Phys Ther.* 2007;87:455-467.

13 Rothstein JM, Echternach JL. *Primer on Measurement: An Introductory Guide to Measurement Issues.* Alexandria, VA: American Physical Therapy Association; 1993.

14 Nilsson BB, Hellesnes B, Westheim A, Risberg MA. Group-based aerobic interval training in patients with chronic heart failure: Norwegian Ullevaal Model. *Phys Ther.* 2008;88:523-535.

15 Fragala-Pinkham MA, Haley SM, Rabin J, Kharasch VS. A fitness program for children with disabilities. *Phys Ther.* 2005;85:1182-1200.

16 Piva SR, Goodnite EA, Azuma K, et al. Neuromuscular electrical stimulation and volitional exercise for individuals with rheumatoid arthritis: a multiple-patient case report. *Phys Ther.* 2007; 87:1064-1077.

Minimal Clinically Important Difference

The minimal clinically important difference (MCID) of a test also is important when deciding if real change has occurred. "Real" in this case means *clinically meaningful* change. Change may be detectable, but is it important? Does it make a worthwhile difference in what a patient is able to do—or not?[6] As Haley and Fragala-Pinkham asked about the change in the child's PEDI mobility scores from 6.1 at admission to 35.9 after 3 weeks, "What do the summary scores from the outcome measures mean? How do we interpret the change score? Has the child achieved 'clinically significant change' up to this point in the hospitalization and physical therapy episode of care? Is the change meaningful?"[6(p736)]

The MCID is defined as the smallest change in the patient's status, as measured by the test, that the patient perceives as beneficial and that could cause a change in the patient's management.[6] Determining what constitutes MCID, however, is not as straightforward as inserting numbers in a mathematical formula. A common way to determine an MCID is to conduct a study using an external criterion or *anchor*.[1] Anchors might be patients, therapists, family members, or others who rate the amount of change that has occurred during an episode of care. This is what Iyer et al[7] did when they assessed the MCID of the PEDI for children in an acute rehabilitation setting, many of whom had acute brain injury. The authors asked clinicians to rate the amount of change that children made and then related the changes to change scores on the PEDI. The researchers determined that the MCID was 8.7 points. The MCID can vary with the patient population, however, so these findings cannot be generalized to all children.[12] The expectation for change in children with acute brain injury, for example, is likely to be much greater than for children with cerebral palsy; therefore, the MCID for children with acute brain injury is likely to be larger than for children with cerebral palsy.

Beninato and colleagues[8] conducted a study to define the MCID for the Functional Independence Measure (FIM) in patients with stroke. They used the change in patients' FIM scores from admission to discharge from a long-term acute care hospital. The anchors were the attending physicians, who rated the patients' change. Based on their ratings, the MCID was 22 for the total FIM, 17 for the motor FIM, and 3 for the cognitive FIM. Less change, therefore, would not be considered clinically important.

Researchers also have identified the MCID for tests that therapists use with patients who have musculoskeletal conditions. Leggin and colleagues,[9] for example, determined the MCID of the Penn Shoulder Score with patients receiving physical therapy for shoulder pain. The anchors in this study were the patients, who rated their pain, satisfaction, and function. The MCID was 11.4 points. If you were writing a case report and used the Penn Shoulder Score as an outcome measurement for a patient similar to those in the study, you could report a clinically important difference if the patient's score improved by 11.4 points or more.

A clinician is treating a patient with subacute low back pain using a novel manual therapy technique and wants to describe the technique and report the patient's outcomes. The clinician routinely assesses pain intensity in his clinic and decides to use the numerical pain rating scale (NPRS) as an outcome measure for the case report.

The NPRS is an 11-point scale, ranging from 0 (no pain) to 10 (worst imaginable pain). The NPRS has been recommended as an accepted outcome measure for pain studies, and change thresholds have been reported for the NPRS.[1] The clinician identified a study that used a global rating-of-change scale as an external criterion to define improved and stable groups of patients with subacute low back pain.[2] This study reported that the MCID for the NPRS was 2 points, meaning that 2 NPRS points was the minimum changed needed to predict differences between the improved and stable groups.[2]

The clinician uses the NPRS at 4 separate times, starting at baseline and ending when the patient is discharged 6 weeks later. The patient's scores show steady progress over the duration of treatment, with NPRS scores exceeding the MCID from baseline to 2 weeks and from 2 weeks to 4 weeks. The scores from 4 weeks to discharge do not exceed the MCID, but the overall change of 7 points from baseline to discharge does exceed the MCID.

	Baseline	2 Weeks	4 Weeks	Discharge
Patient	8	5	2	1

One way to report these patient outcomes is shown here, but this is not the only way. Because this is a case report with no controls, the author does not say that the manual therapy caused the decrease in pain:

The patient had clinically meaningful improvements in pain intensity from baseline to discharge. These improvements appeared to have occurred from baseline to 2 weeks and from 2 weeks to 4 weeks, but not from 4 weeks to discharge. These improvements were believed to be clinically meaningful because they were large enough to distinguish between stable and improved patient groups in a previous study.[2]

References

1 Dworkin RH, Turk DC, Wyrwich KW, et al. Interpreting the clinical importance of treatment outcomes in chronic pain clinical trials: IMMPACT recommendations. J Pain. 2008;9:105-121.

2 Childs JD, Piva SR, Fritz JM. Responsiveness of the numeric pain rating scale in patients with low back pain. Spine. 2005;30:1331-1334.

When the MDC and MCID are available, case report authors should report them and use them to interpret change in scores. If they are not available, authors should explain why they think any measured change was real change and why they think the change was important—if they do. In either case, reliable measurements are important for showing change, and case report authors need to assure readers that their measurements were reliable. (See **Chapter 4**).

What Outcome Measurements Should You Report?

A discussion of measurement in a case report would not be complete without addressing this question. When an author describes the patient's outcome in a case report, the strongest argument the author can make to support the possible value of the patient/client management is to thoroughly describe the changes in the patient's functional activities and participation. Descriptions of changes in body structures and functions (eg, range of motion, force production, pain level) alone should not be used to measure patient outcomes. These measurements may have changed but may not be related to functional gains (ie, may not have concurrent validity with functional ability); activities measured in the clinic may not predict performance at home (ie, may have poor predictive validity). In a case report, it can be important to report changes that relate to patients' body structures and functions—but, as you'll see in the next chapter, in many cases, it is even more important to report changes in activities and participation.

NEXT

Putting Words on Paper

You've chosen your case, thought out your focus, operationalized your definitions, and considered reliability, validity, diagnostic accuracy, and what constitutes real change. Now it's time to write! The hardest part about writing is getting started, and nothing creates writer's block more than when you sit down to begin at the beginning. Words that once flowed so effortlessly through your mind may disappear when you are faced with a blank first page. This manual starts with the introduction because it comes first in the manuscript. But feel free to begin writing wherever you like.

References

1 Elveru RA, Rothstein JM, Lamb RL. Goniometric reliability in a clinical setting: subtalar and ankle measurements. *Phys Ther.* 1988;68:672-677.

2 Youdas JW, Bogard CL, Suman VJ. Reliability of goniometric measurements and visual estimates of ankle joint range of motion obtained in a clinical setting. *Arch Phys Med Rehabil.* 1993;74:1113-1118.

3 Ten Berge SR, Halbertsma JP, Maathuis PG, et al. Reliability of popliteal angle measurement: a study in cerebral palsy patients and healthy controls. *J Pediatr Orthop.* 2007;27:648-652.

4 Kirshner B, Guyatt B. A methodological framework for assessing health and disease. *J Chronic Dis.* 1985;38:27-36.

5 Ottenbacher KJ, Johnson MB, Hojem M. The significance of clinical change and clinical change of significance: issues and methods. *Am J Occup Ther.* 1988;42:156-163.

6 Haley SM, Fragala-Pinkham MA. Interpreting change scores of tests and measures used in physical therapy. *Phys Ther.* 2006;86:735-743.

7 Iyer LV, Haley SM, Watkins MP, Dumas HM. Establishing minimal clinically important differences for scores on the Pediatric Evaluation of Disability Inventory for inpatient rehabilitation. *Phys Ther.* 2003;83:888-898.

8 Beninato M, Gill-Body KM, Salles S, et al. Determination of the minimal clinically important difference in the FIM instrument in patients with stroke. *Arch Phys Med Rehabil.* 2006;87:32-39.

9 Leggin BG, Michener LA, Shaffer MA, Et al. The Penn Shoulder Score: reliability and validity. *J Orthop Sports Phys Ther.* 2006;36:138-151.

PART 2

Start Writing

"Writing is a rough trade.
D'abord, il faut durer.
[Above all, hang in there]."

Ernest Hemingway

"The Introduction": Making the Case for Your Case

Just as mystery writers supply motives for what their characters do, case report writers should supply a rationale for what the therapist does.

Use checklists to keep on track

The introduction, or background and purpose, is the first part of a case report, after the title and abstract (more about titles and abstracts later—they're easier to write once you've written the rest of the case report). In most kinds of case reports, the background and purpose are followed by the case description, which covers the patient history, systems review, examination, evaluation, and intervention (**Chapter 7**); the outcomes section (**Chapter 8**); and the discussion (**Chapter 9**). The content of these sections may change somewhat based on the focus of your case report (see **Chapter 2**). For a detailed checklist of the important components of a case report, refer to the **Appendixes**. Using the checklist will help you keep on track as you write your report.

As in a research paper, the background and purpose of a case report set the stage. Not only do they introduce the topic and focus of the case and explain why the case is important, but they communicate to the reader that there is sufficient support or rationale for the way the case was managed. Clear and credible rationale is needed—regardless of whether the purpose of the report is to describe an unusual case, share information about an intervention, or cast doubt on a theory. The introduction should clearly explain:

- Why the topic is important
- What is known—and not known—about the topic
- The theoretical context for the case, if available
- The support that exists for the management aspects of the case
- The gap in the literature that the case report will fill
- The purpose of the case report

How long should the introduction be? This varies among journals. *PTJ* asks case report authors to not exceed a total of 3,500 words (or about 15 typed double-spaced pages in length). As a rough guideline, allow 800 to 1,000 words for the introduction; 1,500 to 2,000 words for the case description; 250 to 500 words for the outcomes section; and 800 words for the discussion. The actual length of each section will depend, of course, on the amount of material that you need to cover for the purposes and focus of your case report.

Start With Your Knowledge of Practice

Most introductions start by clearly explaining why the topic is an important one. In a case report on an intervention for a patient with chronic lumbar disk extrusion and associated radiculopathy, Hahne and Ford[1] made an immediate, focused argument about the importance of the condition and lack of information on management of patients who have it:

The annual incidence of lumbar disk herniation (LDH) has been estimated to be 1% of the population.[1] When an LDH results in clinical evidence of radiculopathy, and if conservative treatment such as medication and physical therapy fails, diskectomy often is recommended.[1,2] There is no consensus, however, as to the most effective conservative treatment for lumbar disk herniation with associated radiculopathy (LDHR).

In the first few sentences of their introduction, Hahne and Ford accomplished 2 tasks: They gave a rationale for the importance of their topic (a relatively large number of people have the condition and we lack information about effective intervention for it), and they set the stage for their subsequent discussion about research on interventions for people with lumbar disk herniation with or without associated radiculopathy. Next they identified a gap in the research, which was the lack of information about the use of functional restoration programs for people with lumbar disk herniation. To help fill this gap, the purpose of their case report was to describe the use of a functional restoration program with a patient who had chronic lumbar disk extrusion and associated radiculopathy. The authors' approach is clear and direct—and it is likely to capture the attention of readers who work with patients who have similar problems.

The background and justification of your case come in part from your knowledge of practice. That knowledge is shaped by a process of trial and error—as you observe what goes wrong and what works—and by a process of inquiry, which begins when you ask yourself such questions as "Why is there no change with this intervention?" and "Why did this particular way of stretching seem to make such a difference in this patient's pain and function?" The inquiry process continues when you share your observations with colleagues and try to find explanations for what you have seen. But even though sharing anecdotes in the clinic can help stimulate ideas about how to introduce your case, those ideas cannot stand alone.

A Critical Review of the Literature

The trial-and-error process and the intuition of the clinician are extremely important sources of knowledge for understanding practice and for building a foundation for future research. An even more highly valued source of knowledge comes from research using the scientific method.[2] If knowledge derived from trial and error and intuition is to make a meaningful contribution to the professional knowledge base, it must be placed in the context of existing literature—preferably the research literature. A common saying among investigators in many fields is that "one must stand on the shoulders of giants to see farther." The scientific literature provides the "shoulders" on which the evidence base of practice can be built.

Case reports start with a "clinical claim." You've already searched the literature to determine whether your case can contribute something new to the profession; now you must go one step further to find out what is known or not known about your clinical claim. Based on his clinical experience, Alnwick[3] made the following claim in a case report:

> For physical therapists to become more autonomous practitioners and to meet the American Physical Therapy Association goal of Vision 2020,[1] careful examination and evaluation procedures must be used to question the referral diagnosis rather than to blindly proceed with treatment for fibromyalgia and other disorders of the neuromuscular and musculoskeletal systems.

Alnwick did not stop there. He went on to explain and support his claim with knowledge reported in the literature. The literature that he needed to cover is clear from his claim: support for alternative causes of symptoms of patients with a referral diagnosis of fibromyalgia, and support for the components of a differential diagnosis.

Even if you find cases similar to yours in the literature, you may have different outcomes to report or another clinical claim or perspective to offer. In an introduction to multiple-patient case reports, for example, Harris et al[4(p609)] stated, "Although a number of published studies have described neonatal behavioral differences in infants with FAS [fetal alcohol syndrome][3-5] as well as developmental motor outcomes...none of these reports have provided assessment data collected at repeated intervals...." After making this claim, Harris et al had to report the literature describing neonatal behavioral differences and developmental motor outcomes in infants with FAS and the literature supporting the need for repeated assessment data.

In the literature review incorporated into the introduction of a case report on postoperative management of flexor pollicis longus tendon laceration, Ahlschwede[5] provided a table that contained a summary comparison of protocols that had been published in the literature (Table 4). As you'll see in subsequent chapters, tables (and figures) can be a useful way to convey information in case reports.

TABLE 4. Example of a Tabular Summary of Literature Review Findings

No. of Weeks After Repair	Protocol			
	Immobilization	Duran[a]	Kleinert[b]	Washington[c]
1	Immobilization in cast – moderate flexion	Dorsal block splint – wrist 20°, MP 45°, IP neutral, passive ROM to affected digit	Dorsal block splint – wrist 45°, MP 50°, IP relaxed, active extension against traction	Dorsal block splint – wrist 45°, MP 40°, IP 0°, active extension against traction, protected passive ROM to affected digit
3	Discontinue cast, begin active ROM	Continue same	Passive ROM if contracture	Continue same
4	Continue active flexion and extension	Begin active ROM in splint	Allow more wrist extension in splint	Continue same
5	Passive extension as tolerated, no splint	Discontinue splint	Discontinue splint, add wrist cuff	Discontinue traction, full active ROM in splint
6	Dynamic splint for more extension, if needed	Continue active exercise	Unrestricted active ROM	More wrist extension
7	–	–	–	Discontinue splint, allow light use
8	–	Strengthening	Strengthening	Blocking, graded resistance
12	Full, normal activity	Full, normal activity	Full, normal activity	Full, normal activity

Note: MP = metacarpophalangeal joint; IP = intercarpophalangeal joint; ROM = range of motion
[a] (Duran, Houser, Coleman, & Stover, 1984). [b] (Jaeger & MacKin, 1984). [c] (Chow et al., 1987).

Adapted with permission of the American Occupational Therapy Association from Ahlschwede K. Postoperative management of flexor pollicis longus laceration in two cases. Am J Occup Ther. 1991;45:361-365.

You may envision long hours on your computer or in the library trying to uncover everything that has been written on your topic, but that isn't the purpose of a case report's literature review. The introduction should simply provide evidence of the process of inquiry that you used to enhance your understanding of your particular case.

The process of inquiry involves critically reviewing the literature—with the emphasis on critically. Depoy and Gitlin[6] recommended using 3 questions to assist in a critical review of the literature:

1. What work has already been done on this topic or related topics? Is that work relevant to your case?

2. How has the existing knowledge been generated (eg, research versus someone's opinion)? How strong is the evidence for the truth of the knowledge?

3. What theory exists to provide a framework for the case?

Let's look at how these questions may apply in real life. Imagine that you are Dunning and colleagues[7] and that you believe that an intervention approach for a patient with chronic stroke who lacks active write and finger motion is worth reporting. As you prepare to "make your case for your case," you must critically review the literature.

The first step in any literature review is to identify the key topic areas. Depending on the patient's problem, several topics may apply, and there may be a large amount of supporting literature—or no literature at all. Begin by setting some parameters.

> Don't try to cover everything

Dunning et al[7] identified several key topics for their literature review. They started by citing literature to support the importance of stroke as a problem. They then reviewed literature on research to improve upper-extremity function in people with stroke, including research demonstrating the effectiveness of task-specific approaches, such as constraint-induced therapy (CIT). People without wrist and finger movements, however, are not candidates for CIT, so the authors reviewed research supporting the use of neuromuscular electrical stimulation (NMES) to improve active wrist extension to allow a patient to participate in modified CIT. The authors then reviewed the problems associated with the use of NMES and literature that supported the use of a neuroprosthesis combined with task-specific activities for patients with chronic stroke.

Note that these authors covered literature that related directly to their topic. They did not include irrelevant or marginally relevant information. They didn't review the research on the causes of stroke, for example, or even the research on other physical therapy approaches. Although such information is related to the topic, the authors didn't need to include it to achieve their purpose of describing the use of a combination of functional electrical stimulation (with a neuroprosthesis) and task-specific training in a man with chronic stroke who had no active wrist or finger movements.

Again, you don't have to cite every article or book chapter related to your topic, but you should give a fair overview of the most recent and credible work. Identifying the key concepts will help you to develop the rationale for your case, regardless of how much or how little is known. For instance:

- In a case report on joint mobilization for a patient with restricted hip motion following hip resurfacing arthroplasty (HRA), Crow et al[8] provided a "light" review of the literature in their introduction. Their introduction included summary statements from literature about (1) the rationale for the use of resurfacing arthroplasty instead of total hip arthroplasty for younger patients with hip osteoarthritis, (2) what resurfacing arthroplasty involves, and (3) rationale for the use of joint mobilization with patients with restricted motion following HRA. The authors then proceeded to state the purpose of their case report, which was to describe "the treatment for a patient who developed severely restricted hip motion following bilateral HRA."[8(p1592)]

- In a case report of a patient with developmental coordination disorder (DCD), Kaufman and Schilling[9] wrote a relatively "heavy" literature review. First, they provided background information about the problems of children with DCD, including a theory that their incoordination may be due to poor proprioception. Because they knew that some readers might not be familiar with DCD, they reviewed signs and symptoms of DCD, the criteria for a diagnosis of DCD, and controversies in the literature about the underlying deficits. Finally, they reviewed research on interventions for DCD and identified a structured strength training program as a potentially beneficial intervention that researchers had not yet studied.

As you read various journals, note that the extent of the literature review varies among case reports. Remember that, regardless of length, the purpose of the introduction is to provide the rationale and foundation that underlie the purpose of your case report.

Question #2:
How Has the Existing Knowledge Been Generated?

In your search of the literature, have you found case reports, people's opinions, or research? The more credible your sources of information, the more credible your introduction will be. Although case reports and people's opinions can stimulate and provide some support for your ideas, they are not highly credible sources of knowledge. Primary sources of information, particularly research reports, are by far the best sources of knowledge (see **Chapter 3**). Not all research is equal, however; the credibility of research and the ways in which it can be interpreted depend on the type and quality of the research design.

How can a clinician with minimal research background make decisions about the quality of research design during a literature search? Ask yourself this key question: Is the research descriptive or explanatory? Descriptive studies, as explained in **Chapter 1**, disclose existing conditions or examine relationships among variables without manipulating them. Descriptive studies cannot identify cause-and-effect relationships. These studies often use only descriptive statistics (eg, means, standard deviations, frequency, minimum, and maximum) or tests of association (eg, correlation or regression). In interpreting these studies, the following caution for statistics students can be helpful to clinicians as well: Correlation does not equal causality! For instance, just because a study finds a statistically significant negative correlation between body weight and amount of exercise—with people who weigh more doing less exercise than people who weigh less—we can't say that weight causes people to exercise less or that more exercise causes less weight.

Explanatory studies, on the other hand, are experimental studies in which the researcher manipulates the experimental variables while controlling potentially confounding variables. Experimental studies, therefore, can determine cause-and-effect relationships. The strength of the evidence is stronger for studies that randomly assign subjects to intervention and comparison groups than it is for studies that do not use random assignment. You might be able to tell whether a study is explanatory by the types of statistical tests that are used, such as t tests and analyses of variance (ANOVAs).

Another easy way to address the quality of the design without knowing much about research is to answer a related question: Is the study published in a peer-reviewed journal, or is it published in a textbook or a professional magazine or journal that is not peer reviewed? Articles in peer-reviewed journals are critically reviewed both by reviewers who have expertise in the topic area and by journal editors (see **Chapters 3** and **11**). That is not to say that the research published in peer-reviewed journals never has design flaws—most research does. But when an article has passed peer review, you can expect that the flaws are not so serious that they would jeopardize the credibility of the study. As part of your evaluation of the literature, be sure to read the discussion sections of research articles, in which the authors often identify the design flaws for you and discuss how those flaws affect interpretation of the results.

> You *can* judge the quality of the research

In their case report, Kaufman and Schilling[9] cited several journal articles in their review of interventions for children with DCD. Because of the lack of research involving children with DCD, however, support for their intervention had to come from generalizing research on strengthening exercise for children with typical development and from books and review articles. The credibility of the case report would have been stronger if the authors had been able to support their approach with good-quality research articles directly related to their patient group. As is often the case in rehabilitation, however, such research was not available.

When writing your introduction, be sure to clearly differentiate information that is research-based from information that is an opinion or a conclusion. Using such words as "found," "revealed," and "identified" leads the reader to believe that the information is the result of primary research. "Concluded," "believed," and "attributed" are words that suggest the information is not a primary research finding. An author you are citing might have drawn a conclusion or proposed an explanation based on research findings; if this is the case, be sure to say so, to avoid suggesting that the author's conclusion or proposal is an actual research finding when it is not.

This is a subtle but important distinction to convey in writing. Consider an example from a case report by Blanton and Wolf[10(p848)] on the use of upper-extremity constraint-induced movement therapy for a patient with stroke: "Tower[4] noted that following unilateral lesions of the pyramidal tract at the spinal cord level, monkeys would fail to use the affected side." Use of the verb "noted" suggests that Tower made the observation during a research study. On the other hand, the verb "explained" in the following sentence from Blanton and Wolf does not support a primary research finding: "Traub et al[5] explained the learned nonuse behavior as resulting from the animals' inability to move the deafferented extremity due to the presence of a shock-like condition that persists weeks or months after removal of sensory input through all cervical dorsal roots."

Who's Your Audience?

Where do you want to publish? It might seem premature to ask this question, but it's not. Different journals have different audiences and different requirements, and that has a bearing on how you write your case report. Find out which journals publish case reports, then read several reports in each journal to determine whether your case is more like those published in one journal than in another. *PTJ*, for instance, publishes case reports across the broad spectrum of physical therapist practice; other journals might be more specialized. Do the colleagues who could best use your information read one journal more often than another? Would you like to reach an interdisciplinary audience? Could you reach a wider audience by publishing the case report in a journal such as *PTJ* that is indexed in MEDLINE or another database?

Once you have decided on a journal, you can "customize" your report according to the style and readership of that journal. Obtain a copy of the journal's instructions for authors (most journals post those on their Web site), and follow them carefully. Instructions include referencing style, limitations on the number of pages, formats for tables and figures, how to write the cover page, and requirements for the abstract. You can find *PTJ* Information for Authors at *http://www.ptjournal.org/misc/ifora.dtl*.

TABLE 5. An Overview of the *International Classification of Functioning, Disability and Health* (ICF)

	Part 1: Functioning and Disability		Part 2: Contextual Factors	
Components	Body Functions and Structures	Activities and Participation	Environmental Factors	Personal Factors
Domains	Body functions and structures	Life areas (tasks, actions)	External influences on functioning and disability	Internal influences on functioning and disability
Constructs	Change in body functions (physiological) Change in body structures (anatomical)	*Capacity* Executing tasks in a standard environment *Performance* Executing tasks in the current environment	Facilitating or hindering impact of features of the physical, social, and attitudinal world	Impact of attributes of the person
Positive aspect	Functional and structural integrity	Activities Participation	Facilitators	Not applicable
	Functioning			
Negative aspect	Impairment	Activity limitation Participation restriction	Barriers/ hindrances	Not applicable
	Disability			

Adapted with permission of the World Health Organization from International Classification of Functioning, Disability and Health. Geneva, Switzerland: World Health Organization; 2001:11.

The Nagi model describes disability as a linear process in which pathology may progress toward disability, and the IOM model highlights disability as interactions of the individual with environmental conditions. The ICF model moves away from the "consequences of disease" concept to one of "components of health." That is, the objective of the ICF is not to determine causal pathways leading to disablement, but to provide a framework for identifying components of *health* that influence human functioning. Disability and functioning are considered to exist along a continuum of health, as interactive constructs encompassing health condition and contextual factors. The intent is to have a universal language and framework that allow a shared conceptual understanding of health, bridging disciplines, sectors, cultures, and geographic regions.[18,26]

As shown in Table 5, the ICF is divided into 2 parts: (1) functioning and disability, which includes body functions and structures and activities and participation, and (2) contextual factors, which include environmental factors and personal factors. The term "body functions" refers to physiological and psychological mechanisms, whereas "body structures" refers to anatomy. Activities are tasks carried out by an individual, whereas participation is an individual's engagement in a life situation. Environmental factors are external to the individual (eg, physical, social, and attitudinal factors), whereas personal factors consist of the characteristics and life circumstances of the individual.

Body functions and structures may be framed in positive or negative terms.[18] *Functional and structural integrity* denotes functioning in positive terms, whereas anomaly, deviation, or loss in body structure or function is "impairment," a negative term. The ICF doesn't assume that impairment is a fixed health outcome or a static point along the continuum of health. This is because impairments may change through time—they might be progressive or regressive, intermittent or continuous. Impairments might be due to one or multiple health conditions, or the health condition might not fully explain the impairment. In fact, in the ICF, presence of impairment doesn't assume presence of disease. A traumatic amputation of the leg would result in impairment; however, the impairment is not due to a disease or disorder. Impairment might be mild, moderate, severe, or total, and the ICF uses codes with "qualifiers" to indicate the magnitude or extent of the impairment (on a scale of 0-4, 0= indicates no impairment, 1=mild, 2=moderate, 3=severe, and 4=complete or total impairment). Without these qualifiers, the ICF codes have no inherent meaning.

Activities and participation also may be framed in positive or negative terms.[18] *Carrying out activities* and *participating in life situations* describe functioning in positive terms. Activities represent functioning at an individual level, whereas participation represents social functioning. In a negative sense, *activity limitations* refers to difficulties that an individual may have in completing a task. Similarly, *participation restriction* refers to difficulty engaging in life situations. ICF activity and participation classification codes also have qualifiers. A "performance" qualifier describes what an individual does in his or her usual or current environment, whereas a "capacity" qualifier describes what an individual does in a "standardized" environment, that is, an environment supporting functional levels of independence. Both types of qualifiers may apply with or without the use of assisted devices or personal assistance. The difference between performance and capacity indicates the impact of environmental modifications on performance.

Environmental factors might positively or negatively influence body structures and function and activities and participation.[18] The physical, social, and attitudinal elements of the environment may facilitate an individual's performance or create performance barriers. The ICF does not consider personal factors to be part of the health condition but appreciates the influence of individual features (eg, gender and ethnicity) and life circumstance (eg, education and profession) on functioning and disability.

So, functioning and disability are the result of dynamic interactions between an individual's health condition and environmental and personal factors (Figure 15).[18] The ICF does not view disability as an individual attribute, but as a complex relationship between the individual and the social environment. *Functioning* is an umbrella term that covers integrity of body functions and structures, activities, and participation. It describes the positive aspects of the interaction between an individual with a health condition and that individual's contextual factors, specifically environmental and personal factors. *Disability* is an umbrella term that takes into account impairment, activity limitation, and participation restriction.

How does the ICF relate to case reports? By shedding light on the relationships between health conditions and contextual factors, the ICF enables therapists to better understand how and why interventions may have an impact on a patient's ability to function. In fact, case reports are an excellent format for describing intervention designed to improve functioning and for

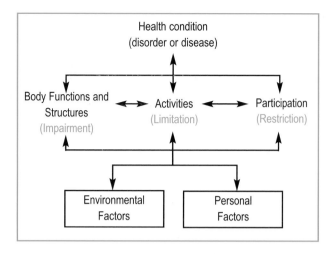

FIGURE 15. Interactions between the components of the *International Classification of Functioning, Disability and Health* (ICF) model.

Reprinted with permission of the World Health Organization from *International Classification of Functioning, Disability and Health*. Geneva, Switzerland: World Health Organization; 2001:18.

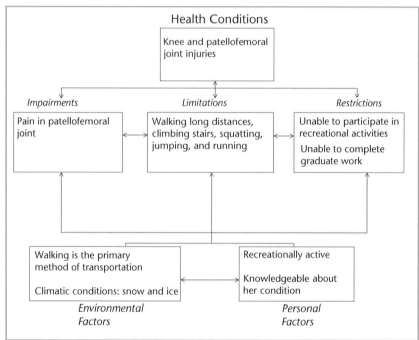

FIGURE 16. Identification of patient information and classification into the *International Classification of Functioning, Disability and Health* framework.

Reprinted from Helgeson K, AR Smith. Process for applying the *International Classification of Functioning, Disability and Health* model to a patient with patellar dislocation. *Phys Ther.* 2008 88:956-964; Figure 2. Modified and reprinted with permission from *International Classification of Functioning, Disability and Health*: ICF. Geneva, Switzerland: World Health Organization; 2001.

describing therapy in relation to disability models and the ICF framework. As Verbrugge and Jette[20] pointed out, communication is made difficult when undefined terms are used to describe the disablement process. By using the ICF framework for clearly describing patient/client management and outcomes, the case report writer provides another set of operational definitions that can help others understand and replicate the case.

Note the way in which Martin et al[27] used the ICF model in their case report of the use of constraint-induced movement therapy with a young child. Helgeson and Smith[28] also applied the ICF in their case report of a patient with patellar dislocation (**Figure 16**). You can find the latter as an annotated case report in **eAppendix 1** (online supplement).

The Hypothesis-Oriented Algorithm for Clinicians II (HOAC II)

The HOAC II[19] provides another framework that could be helpful for organizing the content of a case report. It follows the patient/client management process in the *Guide to Physical Therapist Practice*[25] and includes a detailed step-by-step procedure for any type of patient. The authors designed the HOAC II to be more compatible with contemporary practice than the original HOAC[29] and added the concept of prevention to the framework.

Riddle et al[30] illustrated the application of the HOAC II in their case report of an episode of care of a patient with low back pain. The case report clearly described each step of the HOAC II, from initial data collection through implementation of the intervention and measurement of outcomes (Figure 17). Because some readers might not be familiar with the use of certain terms included in the HOAC II, the authors provided a helpful appendix with definitions at the end of their case report.

The Purpose Statement

The review of related literature should lead clearly and logically to the purpose of the case report, which usually is stated explicitly at the end of the introduction. For their case report about the use of constraint-induced movement therapy (CIMT) with a 3-year-old child with spastic cerebral palsy (CP), Martin et al[27] wrote:

> Previous studies documenting changes in children with hemiplegic CP were not specifically designed to show changes at the multiple levels outlined in the ICF. The purpose of this case study was to explore changes associated with a CIMT trial on a child's function at all ICF Levels of Activity and Participation and Body Structure and Function, as identified by (1) parent-identified occupation goals of participation and activities, (2) quality of upper-extremity movement, (3) performance of self-care skills, and (4) grip and pinch strength with a 3-year-old child. By measuring the child's performance simultaneously at the different levels, the intent was to identify possible associations between body structure and function and activity and participation changes.

A good introduction leads readers so directly to the purpose statement that they can guess the purpose of the case report before reading it.

NEXT

Who (or What) Is Your Focus?

The purpose statement helps to focus readers' attention as they begin to read the next section—the case description. Of all the components of the case report, this may be the one that comes easiest to you, because often it focuses on what therapists know best: the patient.

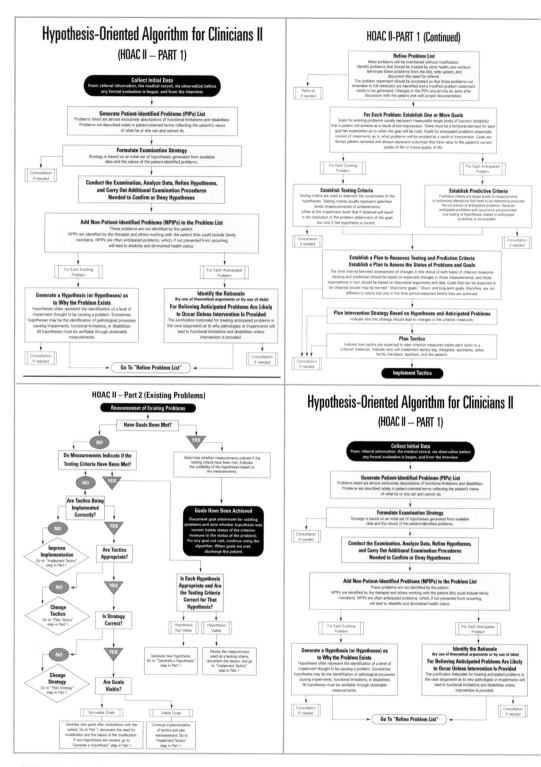

FIGURE 17. Riddle et al[30] illustrated the application of the HOAC II in their case report of an episode of are of a patient with low back pain, from initial data collection through implementation of the intervention and measurement of outcomes.

Reprinted from Riddle DL, Rothstein JM, Echternach JL. Application of the HOAC II: an episode of care for a patient with low back pain. *Phys Ther.* 2003;83:471-485; Figures 1-4.

Chapter 6: "The Introduction": Making the Case for Your Case

References

1 Hahne AJ, Ford JJ. Functional Restoration for a chronic lumbar disk extrusion with associated radiculopathy. *Phys Ther.* 2006;86:1668-1680.

2 Portney LG, Watkins MP. *Foundations of Clinical Research: Applications to Practice.* 3rd ed. Upper Saddle River, NJ: Prentice Hall; 2009.

3 Alnwick GM. Misdiagnosis of serotonin syndrome as fibromyalgia and the role of physical therapists. *Phys Ther.* 2008;88:757-765.

4 Harris S, Osborn J, Weinberg J, et al. Effects of prenatal alcohol exposure on neuromotor and cognitive development during early childhood: a series of case reports. *Phys Ther.* 1993;73:608-617.

5 Ahlschwede K. Postoperative management of flexor pollicis longus laceration in two cases. *Am J Occup Ther.* 1991;45:361-365.

6 Depoy E, Gitlin LN. *Introduction to Research Understanding and Applying Multiple Strategies.* 3rd ed. St Louis, MO: CV Mosby Co; 2005.

7 Dunning K, Berberich A, Albers B, et al. A 4our-week, task-specific neuroprosthesis program for a person with no active wrist or finger movement because of chronic stroke. *Phys Ther.* 2008;88:397-405.

8 Crow JB, Gelfand B, Su EP. Use of joint mobilization in a patient with severely restricted hip motion following bilateral hip resurfacing arthroplasty. *Phys Ther.* 2008;88:1591-1600.

9 Kaufman LB, Schilling DL. Implementation of a strength training program for a 5-year-old child with poor body awareness and developmental coordination disorder. *Phys Ther.* 2007;87:455-467.

10 Blanton S, Wolf SL. An application of upper-extremity constraint-induced movement therapy in a patient with subacute stroke. *Phys Ther.* 1999;79:847-853.

11 Korobov S. Developing theory in a practice profession. *Physiother Res Int.* 2007;12:225-227.

12 Krebs DE, Harris SR, Herdman SJ, Michels E. Theory in physical therapy. *Phys Ther.* 1986;66:661-662.

13 Shepard K. Theory: criteria, importance, and impact. In: Lister MJ, ed. *Contemporary Management and Motor Control Problems: Proceedings of the II STEP Conference.* Alexandria, VA: Foundation for Physical Therapy; 1991:5-10.

14 Malouin F, Potvin M, Prévost J, et al. Use of an intensive task-oriented gait training program in a series of patients with acute cerebrovascular accidents. *Phys Ther.* 1992;72:781-788.

15 Lott DJ, Maluf KS, Sinacore DR, Mueller MJ. Relationship between changes in activity and plantar ulcer recurrence in a patient with diabetes mellitus. *Phys Ther.* 2005;85:579-588.

16 McClure PW, Flowers KR. Treatment of limited shoulder motion: a case study based on biomechanical consideration. *Phys Ther.* 1992;72:929-936.

17 Kaltenborn FM. *Mobilization of the Extremity Joints.* Oslo, Norway: Olaf Norlis Bokhandel Universitetsgaten; 1980.

18 *International Classification of Functioning, Disability and Health.* Geneva, Switzerland: World Health Organization; 2001.

19 Rothstein JM, Echternach JL, Riddle DL. The Hypothesis-Oriented Algorithm for Clinicians II (HOAC II): a guide for patient management. *Phys Ther.* 2003;83:455-470.

20 Verbrugge LM, Jette AM. The disablement process. *Soc Sci Med.* 1994;38:1-14.

21 Brandt EN Jr, Pope AM, eds. *Enabling America: Assessing the Role of Rehabilitation Science and Engineering.* Washington, DC: National Academy Press; 1997.

22 Jette AM. Physical disablement concepts for physical therapy research and practice. *Phys Ther.* 1994;74:380-386.

23 Nagi SZ. Some conceptual issues in disability and rehabilitation. In: Sussman MB, ed. *Sociology and Rehabilitation.* Washington, DC: American Sociological Association; 1965:100-113.

24 *National Advisory Board on Medical Rehabilitation Research, Draft V: Report and Plan for Medical Rehabilitation Research.* Bethesda, MD: National Institutes of Health; 1992.

25 *Guide to Physical Therapist Practice.* 2nd ed. *Phys Ther.* 2001;81:9-746.

26 Jette AM. Toward a common language for function, disability, and health. *Phys Ther.* 2006;86:726-734.

27 Martin A, Burtner PA, Poole J, Phillips J. Case report: ICF-level changes in a preschooler after constraint-induced movement therapy. *Am J Occup Ther.* 2008;62:282-288.

28 Helgeson K, Smith AR Jr. Process for applying the International Classification of Functioning, Disability and Health model to a patient with patellar dislocation. *Phys Ther.* 2008;88:956-964.

29 Rothstein JM, Echternach JL. Hypothesis-oriented algorithm for clinicians. *Phys Ther.* 1986;66:1388-1394.

30 Riddle DL, Rothstein JM, Echternach JL. Application of the HOAC II: an episode of care for a patient with low back pain. *Phys Ther.* 2003;83: 471-485.

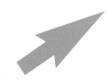

DIAGNOSIS

Both a process and a label. Process includes integrating and evaluating examination data, which the physical therapist organizes into defined clusters, syndromes, or categories to help determine the prognosis (including the plan of care) and the most appropriate intervention strategies. Physical therapists use diagnostic labels that identify the impact of a condition on functioning at the level of the system (especially the movement system) and at the level of the whole person.

PROGNOSIS
(Including Plan of Care)

Determination of the level of optimal improvement that may be attained through intervention and the amount of time required to reach that level. The plan of care specifies the interventions to be used and their timing and frequency.

EVALUATION

A dynamic process in which the physical therapist makes clinical judgments based on data gathered during the examination. This process also may identify possible problems that require consultation with or referral to another provider.

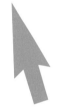

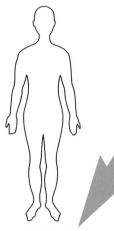

INTERVENTION

Purposeful and skilled interaction of the physical therapist with the patient/client and, if appropriate, with other individuals involved in care of the patient/client, using various physical therapy procedures and techniques to produce changes in the condition that are consistent with the diagnosis and prognosis. The physical therapist conducts a reexamination to determine changes in patient/ client status and to modify or redirect intervention. The decision to reexamine may be based on new clinical findings or on lack of patient/client progress. The process of reexamination also may identify the need for consultation with or referral to another provider.

EXAMINATION

The process of obtaining a history, performing a systems review, and selecting and administering tests and measures to gather data about the patient/client. The initial examination is a comprehensive screening and specific testing process that leads to a diagnostic classification. The examination process also may identify possible problems that require consultation with or referral to another provider.

OUTCOMES

Intended results of patient/client management, which include the impact of physical therapy interventions in the following domains: body functions and structures, activities and participation, environmental factors, and personal factors.

FIGURE 18. The 5 elements of patient/client management.

Adapted with permission of the American Physical Therapy Association from Guide to Physical Therapist Practice. 2nd ed. *Phys Ther.* 2001;81:43.

history of a child with cerebral palsy, the record of a patient's performance on every item of a comprehensive test of activities of daily living (ADL), or the use of a dozen orthopedic tests is not necessary.

As part of the operational definition of the patient history, systems review, and other components of their examination, authors should clarify for the reader the sources of data reported in the case report. Remember that one goal of your description is "replicability." After reading your case report, other therapists with similar professional experience should be able to collect the same type of information about a patient with a similar problem.

A good way to avoid omitting important steps in the clinical process is to follow a guide for patient/client management. Depending on the target audience for your case report, the *Guide to Physical Therapist Practice*,[2] the *Guide to Occupational Therapy Practice*,[3] or the *Occupational Therapy Practice Framework*[4] would be good sources of information about processes and terminology as they have been described and defined by the American Physical Therapy Association and the American Occupational Therapy Association, respectively. Figure 18 defines the 5 elements of patient/client management from the *Guide to Physical Therapist Practice*.[2] Figure 19 illustrates the occupational therapy process.[4] Although the terminology and emphases differ somewhat, the overall processes are similar.

When It's About Your Patient: The History

In case reports involving people, the first subheading in the case description usually is "Patient," "Client," "Child," "Student," or another term that is appropriate for the case. The patient description often includes such information as age, sex, history, and any other relevant background information that could have contributed or did contribute to the clinical reasoning process. In the *Guide to Physical Therapist Practice*,[2] this type of information is included in the patient/client history; in the *Occupational Therapy Practice Framework*,[4] this information is included in the occupational profile part of the evaluation.

The patient is a common source of information. Other sources may include the patient's physician, the patient's family or friends, and the patient's medical chart. Figure 20 gives a comprehensive list of the types of information that may be obtained in taking a history. Obviously, not all of the information is relevant for all patients. An important contribution of a case report is to show what pieces of information are important for particular patients with particular characteristics and how that information informs the decision-making process.

Be sure to say why you chose this patient for the case report, especially when the case is not unusual. For instance, were particular patients with carpal tunnel syndrome selected because they got better and others did not? Unless the patient is obviously unusual or unique, clearly state your selection criteria. When describing more than one patient, describe the first patient thoroughly, adding only important differences for the other patients.[5] Throughout the description, be careful to disguise patient identity, even though you have the patient's permission to write the case report.

Uncertainty is a fact of life in clinical practice; the case report is an opportunity to describe how to reduce that uncertainty.

In most published case reports dealing with patients, the patient and the interview data are described in the text of the report; however, as shown by examples later in this chapter, tables and figures also can be useful when the history is lengthy or complex.

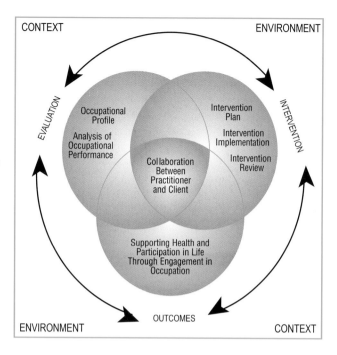

FIGURE 19. The occupational therapy process.

Adapted with permission of the American Occupational Therapy Association from Roley SS, DeLany JV, Barrows CJ, et al. Occupational therapy practice framework: domain and process. 2nd ed. *Am J Occup Ther.* 2008;62:625-683; Figure 2.

The patient's symptoms, reason for seeking care, and desired outcomes typically are included, using descriptions that delineate the patient's activity limitations and participation restrictions. History information that is considered to be relevant also should be reported, including a chronologically based description of symptoms.

Patient's Reason for Seeking Care

The interview data reported by Crow et al [6(p1592)] elucidated the patient's reason for seeking care (he was diagnosed with osteoarthritis and had a hip resurfacing arthroplasty [HRA]) and indicated the extent of the patient's activity limitations and participation restrictions:

> The patient was a 43-year-old, athletic man who underwent bilateral HRA secondary to severe OA. He had a long history of bilateral hip pain and attributed the arthritis to playing football and weight lifting as a youngster. He described a constant, sharp, acute pain in his left hip and a constant dull pain in his right hip. The patient was limited in his activities of daily living (ADL) due to pain and decreased hip ROM. He was limited in donning his socks and shoes, was unable to walk more than a few city blocks or ascend more than one flight of stairs, and could sit only about 5 minutes. Lastly, he stopped all recreational sports and activities due to pain and lack of ROM. Formerly, he had participated in tennis, golf, cycling, and weight lifting.

Similarly, Bellamy et al [7(p141)] described the impairments, activity limitations, and participation restrictions reported by their patient with a diagnosis of multiple pterygium syndrome, a rare genetic disorder that causes connective tissue webbing across joints:

> The client received his first referral to physical therapy when he was 13 years of age. The client's expressed goals for therapy were to improve the cosmesis and mobility of his left knee,

General Demographics
- Age
- Sex
- Race/ethnicity
- Primary language
- Education

Social History
- Cultural beliefs and behaviors
- Family and caregiver resources
- Social interactions, social activities, and support systems

Employment/Work (Job/School/Play)
- Current and prior work (job/school/play), community, and leisure actions, tasks, or activities

Growth and Development
- Developmental history
- Hand dominance

Environment
- Devices and equipment (eg, assistive, adaptive, orthotic, protective, supportive, prosthetic)
- Environment and community characteristics
- Projected discharge destinations

General Health Status (Self-Report, Family Report, Caregiver Report)
- General health perception
- Physical functioning (eg, mobility, sleep patterns, restricted bed days)
- Psychological functioning (eg, memory, reasoning ability, depression, anxiety)
- Participation (roles) (eg, community, leisure, social, work)
- Participation (social) (eg, social activity, social interaction, social support)

Social/Health Habits (Past and Current)
- Behavioral health risks (eg, smoking, drug abuse)
- Level of physical fitness

Family History
- Familial health risks

Medical/Surgical History
- Cardiovascular
- Endocrine/metabolic
- Gastrointestinal
- Genitourinary
- Gynecological
- Integumentary
- Musculoskeletal
- Neuromuscular
- Obstetrical
- Prior hospitalizations, surgeries, and preexisting medical and other health-related conditions
- Psychological
- Pulmonary

Current Condition(s)/Chief Complaint(s)
- Concerns that led the patient/client to seek the services of a physical therapist
- Concerns or needs of patient/client who requires the services of a physical therapist
- Current therapeutic interventions
- Mechanisms of injury or disease, including date of onset and course of events
- Onset and pattern of symptoms
- Patient/client, family, significant other, and caregiver expectations and goals for the therapeutic intervention
- Patient/client, family, significant other, and caregiver perceptions of patient's/client's emotional response to the current clinical situation
- Previous occurrence of chief complaint(s)
- Prior therapeutic interventions

Level of Activity and Participation
- Current and prior activity and participation in self-care and home management, including activities of daily living (ADL) and instrumental activities of daily living (IADL)
- Current and prior activity and participation in work (job/school/play), community, and leisure actions, tasks, or activities

Medications
- Medications for current condition
- Medications previously taken for current condition
- Medications for other conditions

Other Clinical Tests
- Laboratory and diagnostic tests
- Review of available records (eg, medical, education, surgical)
- Review of other clinical findings (eg, nutrition and hydration)

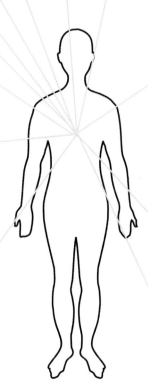

FIGURE 20. Types of data that may be generated from the history. For the purposes of a case report, include only the information that influenced your clinical decision making or that you believe may have had an effect on the outcomes.

Adapted with permission of the American Physical Therapy Association from Guide to Physical Therapist Practice. 2nd ed. *Phys Ther.* 2001;81:44.

to decrease his knee and back pain, to be able to play basketball during gym class, and to be able to walk, not ride in a wheelchair, the next time he went to his favorite theme park.

Sometimes people seek care for another person. Dunbar[8(p227)] described a child's behaviors that led others in the child's environment to refer her for occupational therapy:

The teacher reported that Sara had frequent tantrums and was unable to maintain attention to tabletop tasks. She threw toys at other children and frequently ran around the room when the teacher asked her to stay in her chair. Sara's mother reported that Sara exhibited daring behaviors in the home setting, including jumping from high counters and purposely running into walls. The speech-language pathologist treating Sara for expressive language delays in the school setting recommended occupational therapy to enhance Sara's ability to tolerate the school environment.

History of Other Interventions

Many patients, particularly those with lengthy or chronic problems, have a history of intervention before the episode of care that is the focus of the case report. Did your patient previously receive therapy? If so, describe the intervention as clearly as you can. If the information is based on patient report, that's fine; just be sure to state the source of your information, regardless of what or who it is. Similarly, be sure to report previous medications, surgery, or other interventions, along with the patient's opinion of their effectiveness.

Chronology

A case report written by Ellenbecker et al[9] illustrates the importance of clear chronology when describing the temporal elements of a patient's problem. The authors' purpose was to describe "the detailed rehabilitation program and outcome of a patient who [had] an initial glenohumeral dislocation, followed by multiple surgical interventions prior to shoulder hemiarthroplasty with biologic glenoid resurfacing."[9(p278)] The description of the patient's condition as it changed over time helps other clinicians identify patients with similar characteristics[9(pp277-278)]:

The patient was a 28-year-old male laborer who originally dislocated his dominant right shoulder while playing football at the age of 16. After the initial dislocation, the patient saw a local orthopaedic surgeon and immediately underwent an arthroscopic labral repair. The patient was subsequently able to return to full activity. Three years later the patient underwent a second arthroscopic surgical procedure for recurrent shoulder dislocation secondary to trauma. Observations made by the surgeon during the second surgical procedure included the presence of a posterior labral tear with detachment, a redundant anterior/inferior capsule, a severely stretched middle glenohumeral ligament, a loose body, and early degenerative changes of the humeral articular surface. Surgical debridement chondroplasty was performed, along with removal of the loose body, and an arthroscopic anterior capsulolabral reconstruction.

Following the second surgical procedure, the patient was able to return to some level of functional activity for a period of 7 years. Specifically, he was able to return to sport activities, which included cycling and limited overhead sports, as well as repetitive overhead work activity and work-related lifting. However, he incurred an injury at work that resulted in another glenohumeral joint dislocation. Over the next 2 years, the patient underwent 4 additional surgical procedures, including an arthroscopic subacromial decompression and capsular shift, an open Bankart with repeat capsular shift, an arthroscopic anterior capsular reconstruction with laser chondroplasty for diagnoses of recurrent anterior dislocation and progressive glenohumeral arthritis, and a posterior capsular reconstruction with thermal capsulorrhaphy for a diagnosis of recurrent posterior dislocation. The patient was seen by an orthopaedic surgeon (D.S.B.) 1 year following the last procedure, because of continued pain and reduced shoulder function. At the time of the initial examination the patient had been unable to work at his preinjury level for the previous 5 years and had an active worker's compensation claim. The specific work-related activities that he was unable to perform were heavy lifting, repetitive overhead lifting, and overhead arm positioning.

In this description of a 12-year history, the reader is able to clearly follow the temporal sequence of the patient's condition and interventions. The progressive nature of the impairments and activity limitations also is described clearly.

When describing the temporal sequence of events in a case report, authors typically have used 2 strategies. The first—as used by Ellenbecker and colleagues above—is to reference health-related events to the amount of time passed since the onset of the problem or the current episode of care. The other strategy is to give dates of important health-related historical events that are associated with the patient's condition. The first strategy is preferable. Chronology is easier to grasp when the case report notes the amount of time since the most relevant event (eg, injury or referral for therapy) rather than reporting the dates and requiring the reader to calculate time between events.

Dunbar[8(p232)] explained the chronology of concern about the child in her case report in this way: "The mother reported that Sara was always an active child and that she did not suspect that Sara's behavior was unusual until Sara entered a preschool program.... Sara had attended preschool for approximately 6 months before the referral to occupational therapy. Her mother reported that the teacher had expressed concerns from the first month."

Perhaps the best way to determine whether you have captured the chronology of your case report is to have a colleague read the report. Your colleague should be able to report back to you the temporal sequence of the pertinent events prior to and after referral for therapy.

Systems Review

The systems review is defined by the *Guide to Physical Therapist Practice* as "a brief or limited examination of (1) the anatomical or physiological status of the cardiovascular/pulmonary, integumentary, musculoskeletal, and neuromuscular systems and (2) the communication ability, affect, cognition, language, and learning style of the patient."[2(p42)] The findings of the systems review should be noted and, based on the data obtained so far, the case report should explain how the data helped guide the selection of specific tests and measures and identified possible health problems that might require consultation with or referral to another health care provider.

Vaughn and Nitsch[10(p1580)] focused on the neuromuscular systems in their systems review of a patient with a 2-week history of right low back pain:

> Based on the location of pain, the complaint that the right leg felt longer than the left leg, and her symptoms aggravated by her 2-handed backstroke and right hip extension, the patient's primary problem was believed to be related to SIJD. Screening of the lumbar spine was performed to rule out a neurological dysfunction. This screening included myotome testing of L2–S1, reflex testing of L4 and S1, sensory testing of the lower extremities for crude touch and pinprick, and passive mobility testing.[36] The screening of the lumbar spine was negative for a neurological dysfunction. No structural abnormalities or mobility impairments were identified when screening the ankles, knees, and feet.

In his case report of a patient with a referral diagnosis of fibromyalgia, the patient's interview data and other history led Alnwick[11(p760)] to do a more thorough systems review:

> **Vital signs.** Vital signs were not noted at the time of the initial visit.
>
> **Neurologic findings.** Deep tendon reflexes were grossly 2 in bilateral upper extremities (biceps, triceps, and brachioradialis). Patellar and Achilles tendon reflexes were unattainable bilaterally. Nystagmus of greater than 3 beats was observed bilaterally, along with increased dizziness with finger tracking. The patient had difficulty when she was asked to touch her finger to her nose and then to touch my finger. Sensation to light touch was within normal limits, except for hypersensitivity to very light touch in the entire right lower extremity.
>
> **Musculoskeletal findings.** Palpation revealed tenderness in a nonanatomic pattern throughout the patient's extremities and body. These findings did not coincide with the criteria for fibromyalgia.[3] Because of the patient's increased pain level, a proper assessment of gross range of motion and strength (force-generating capacity) was not performed. The patient's roommate reported that she spent much of the night "jumping" and having muscle spasms with jerking motions in all parts of her body. This problem severely limited her ability to sleep for more than 2 hours at a time.
>
> **Cardiovascular, endocrinologic, and integumentary findings.** There were no significant findings for the cardiovascular, endocrinologic, and integumentary systems.
>
> **Gastrointestinal tract findings.** The patient reported gastrointestinal tract symptoms (nausea, vomiting, and difficulty with bowel and bladder functions).

Chapter 7: Describing the Patient or Other Entity

Other findings. At the time of the initial evaluation, the patient completed and scored 70% on the Oswestry Disability Index (ODI) questionnaire ....The patient's balance was poor, as demonstrated by her need to hold on to a table with both hands in order to remain in an upright position in response to light pressure placed upon her shoulders and torso by the therapist in various directions while she was sitting. Gait assessment demonstrated a severe antalgic gait with the use of a straight cane. The patient also exhibited decreased stride length and stance phase bilaterally with a step-to-gait pattern. She reported that there were times when her legs would "give out" without any apparent warning. This problem had led her to have several recent falls.

Based on the systems review and other examination findings that were not consistent with fibromyalgia, the physical therapist suspected serotonin syndrome as the cause of the patient's problems. He referred the patient back to her primary care physician with a recommendation for referral to a neurologist, who subsequently diagnosed serotonin syndrome.

Make your clinical reasoning explicit

Clinical Impression

To augment the discussion of their clinical reasoning and help make it more explicit for the reader, *PTJ* now asks authors to explain their "clinical impressions" throughout the case report.[12] The initial clinical impression should appear right after the patient history and systems review. The clinical impression brings together information obtained from the history, identifies what the authors believe to be the primary problem or problems at this point, and explains the differential diagnoses to be addressed in the examination.[12] It also should include any other information you need but have not yet obtained and a statement of why you think, at this point, that the patient is a good candidate for the purpose of the case report. For more information about clinical impressions, see information for authors of case reports at *http://www.ptjournal.org/misc/ifora.dtl#Case_Reports*.

An example of an initial clinical impression appears in a case report of 2 patients with traumatic brain injury by Mossberg et al[13(pp79-80)]:

Both patients had characteristics typical of the individual recovering from TBI and were considered good candidates to receive the examination and intervention procedures. Each patient had cognitive impairments but was considered above the minimal requirements needed to perform each of the physical examination procedures reliably. Because of the nature of the injury, further specific tests that integrated all of the major systems were necessary (see "Examination" section). These tests included measures of balance, gait speed, and endurance. Both patients were capable of ambulating over ground without manual assistance at a self-selected speed that consequently allowed for measurements of their gait speed and endurance.

Because both patients were essentially sedentary and had a TBI with residual neuromusculoskeletal impairments, we were interested in a more detailed assessment of their endurance levels. Neither patient exhibited overt cardiovascular, neuromuscular, or musculoskeletal pathology that would have prevented them from performing a peak aerobic capacity test or from participating in a vigorous exercise program. The only concern was possible exercise-induced asthma in patient 2. We always ensured that the patient had her inhaler in her possession when participating in the examination and intervention procedures.

In the examination section that followed, Mossberg and colleagues then described the measurements that, in their clinical impression, they had justified using.

Cahalin et al[14] provide clinical impressions throughout their case report on suspected statin-induced respiratory muscle myopathy during long-term inspiratory muscle training in a patient with diaphragmatic paralysis. They state an initial clinical impression...

> The clinical decision-making process used to select the below-mentioned tests and measures for the patient was based on progressive [dyspnea on exertion]; pulmonary function test (PFT) results revealing a mild to moderate restrictive lung disorder based on the FEV1, FVC, and FEV1/FVC; chest radiograph consistent with right hemidiaphragmatic paralysis; a paradoxical breathing pattern; ABG analysis identifying mild hypoxia[18]; and limited gardening due to DOE during gardening tasks and bending. The [dyspnea on exertion], right hemidiaphragmatic paralysis, and mild hypoxia warranted the examination of the strength (force-generating capacity) and endurance of the inspiratory muscles. Thus, the clinical impression of the patients problems was one of impaired ventilation and respiration/gas exchange associated with ventilatory pump dysfunction.[19]

... as well as provide an impression directly following the examination section:

> These examination findings supported the initial clinical impression of impaired ventilation and respiration/gas exchange associated with ventilatory pump dysfunction,[19] as the [pulmonary function test] results revealed a restrictive lung disorder combined with decreased [inspiratory muscle performance] that resulted in pronounced dyspnea and fatigue. The lower-than-expected [peak inspiratory muscle pressure] PImax, [sustained] PImax, and inspiratory work/endurance identified the ventilatory pump dysfunction and provided a baseline measure from which to develop the plan of care, which included high-intensity [inspiratory muscle training] via the [Test of Incremental Respiratory Endurance, or TIRE] and patient education about [inspiratory muscle training]. All baseline measurements of IMP were reduced, but the measure of inspiratory work/endurance identified the patients inability to complete the TIRE protocol due to very poor inspiratory muscle endurance (Fig. 3) The RT2 TIRE system was used to perform high-intensity [inspiratory muscle training] because it provided the serial presentation of submaximal isokinetic profiles at 80% of MVC within a progressive work-to-rest ratio, with rest periods decreasing from 60 seconds to 5 seconds. Currently, the RT2 TIRE system used with this patient has limited availability. However, standard examination of inspiratory muscle strength... and endurance ... would provide potentially useful information regarding IMP and the possibility of a respiratory muscle [statin-induced skeletal myopathies].

PTJ started requiring explicit clinical impressions in 2007, so few examples exist in its published case reports as this manual goes to press. Here is a fictional example—based on the history and systems review of a truck driver who had posterior thigh pain and intermittent low back pain—that emphasizes the thought process of the physical therapists as they rule in and rule out diagnoses:

Chapter 7: Describing the Patient or Other Entity

The "Nonpatient"

Case reports that deal with entities other than patients (eg, administrative issues) also should describe the entity clearly, include all pertinent information, and reveal the sources of all data. There is a wide variety of cases, and it is not possible to give guidelines for describing all of the possible entities, but you should use the same general guidelines that apply to case reports on patients: Describe the case in such detail that the reader could recognize it or identify similar cases.

When describing a clinical practice, for example, it may or may not be important to describe such diverse characteristics as the square footage of the department, the salary of employees, the elements of the quality improvement program, the program goals, the years of experience therapists have had, the number of patients seen daily, the ethnic makeup of the department staff, or the status of therapist-administrator relations. In general, identify and report the characteristics and information that went into decision making and that could be related to outcomes, regardless of the type of entity being described.

Hazari's case report on the design and implementation of a local area network (LAN)[1] describes a university program:

Over the past 5 years computers had been regularly installed to support instruction. All labs and department offices within the school had their own workstations and peripherals. With a critical need to exchange data, share expensive resources such as plotters and printers, and communicate using electronic mail, it was only a matter of time before the need for a LAN was identified.

It was determined that the network would help support the school's long-term goals as outlined in the Strategic Plan, which emphasized distinction in undergraduate education, plus excellence in teaching, research, and creative activity. Priorities for Action in the plan called for integrating information technology in courses to improve learning.

The case report goes on to describe other characteristics of the program and how they related to the decisions that were made about the LAN's design and implementation. The information about the Strategic Plan and Priorities for Action is an example of the type of detail that could be important information for others trying to develop a similar system.

References

1 Hazari S. Multi-protocol LAN design and implementation: a case study. Technological Horizons in Education Journal. 1995;22(9):80-85.

Because the patient had not had a recent history of LBP, because there were no neurological symptoms such as loss of sensation or parasthesias, because the MRI results were negative, and because he had no pain below the knee, we did not believe at this time that the problem was likely to be from a radiculopathy. Nevertheless, a lower-quarter screening examination would be appropriate to rule in or rule out this possibility.

Because the types of activities that seemed to reproduce symptoms were related to trunk flexion combined with hip and knee extension and moving out of these positions reduced the pain, we hypothesized that the problem may be related to some type of adaptive shortening of soft tissue structures that could limit the patient's ability to flex the trunk and hip and extend the knee simultaneously. Potential shortened structures could be the hamstring muscles or the connective tissues associated with the lumbar spinal nerve roots or sciatic nerve. These tissues might have become adaptively shortened in response to the previous episodes of low back injury and pain. We decided that our examination also should include tests to rule in or rule out these possibilities.

Tests and Measures

When the focus of a case report is a patient or client, the "tests and measures" section begins with an analysis of the information obtained from the interview, chart, other sources of initial data, and the systems review. Based on this information, the therapist selects procedures that are most likely to shed light on the patient's problem (see **Chapters 4 and 5** for more about measurement). If the focus of the report is a clinic, an education program, or another "nonpatient" entity, the analysis will vary. But regardless of the type of case report, you should clearly explain not only what you did to examine the problem, but why you did it. Clinical decisions are difficult to put into words because many times these decisions seem almost reflexive. Nonetheless, the decision-making process must be made explicit for the reader.

> The literature shows that effective practitioners collect only the data they need for deciding what to do next.

The literature shows that effective practitioners collect only the data they need for deciding what to do next. Elstein and colleagues[15] and Payton[16] demonstrated that, early on, when taking the history, clinicians determine what problems are important, what types of examination data are needed, and what interventions may be useful.

Linking Patient Information With the Examination

Excerpts from a published case report show how a clinician focused the examination—directly and indirectly—on the history, symptoms, and goals.

Beattie[17] reported on the management of a patient with low back pain who was unable to compete in a pole vault competition. Beattie clearly linked his approach to the patient's history and goals and decided, based on the location of symptoms and the movements associated with the problematic activity, that spinal motion should be examined:

> The patient's complaints were most noticeable during the take-off phase of pole vaulting. This activity requires that the individual assume a position of spinal extension, with side-bending and rotation of the trunk to the right.[2] The central location of the patient's pain and stiffness suggested that "local" limitation of spinal movement[16] (ie, limited motion in the midlumbar spinal segments) may have been related to his inability to pole vault. Thus, the initial problem statement was that the patient's midlumbar symptoms were associated with an abnormality of spinal motion, which prevented him from pole vaulting.

Most of the data collected during the course of a patient's care are obtained for a reason. Therapists do not have time to do a complete systems review or to measure everything that can be measured during a patient's course of care—nor would they want to do so, because that information would be of little or no use for the decisions they have to make.

When writing a case report, explain why you examined each system or performance component, why you used each test and measure, and what the information from each test and measure contributed to your clinical reasoning. A laundry list of tests and measures, without an explanation of why you did them or what they contributed, is a sure way to get a response from journal reviewers or an instructor saying that the clinical reasoning in your case report is not clear.

Operational Definitions Again!

Operational definitions of the procedures that were used to obtain examination data also must be included in case reports. (Refer to **Chapter 4** for more on operational definitions.) Operational definitions can be accomplished in a variety of ways. Some authors have operationally defined the procedures that they used, whereas others have referenced the operational definitions that were used and published by others. Beattie[17] used a combination:

> The patient's AROM [active range of motion] was normal, as defined by Magee[25] and Hoppenfeld.[26] The straight-leg-raising (SLR) test was performed as described by Hoppenfeld.[26] The patient's SLR was 90 degrees bilaterally, and no pain was elicited during this procedure. Manual muscle testing was performed using the "break test" by requesting the patient to perform each of the eight movements against manual resistance that I applied.[29] No muscular force deficits were noted in the lower extremities. I performed sensory testing, using a light brushing motion with my hands over the dermatomes that correspond to L2 through S2, to determine the presence and symmetry of the patient's light touch sensation.[25,26]
>
> Palpation of the posterior trunk was performed as follows. The patient lay on a treatment table in the prone position. The paravertebral soft tissues were examined using fingertip palpation. Pain was elicited with palpation unilaterally, 1 cm to the right of the spinal segmental levels of L2-4....

Fergus and colleagues[18(p272)] used operational definitions (Table 6) for their video analysis of upper extremity (UE) function in the examination of a child with hemiparesis:

> At 13 months of age, video analysis of the quality and quantity of movement was performed (see Table 1). The child maintained her right UE in a flexion pattern of at least 90° in the proximal interphalangeal joints for 81.4% of the 46-minute observation session. She reached for objects with her right UE 8.9% of the 74 trials when objects were presented at midline. She grasped successfully with the right hand 49.2% of attempts with 3.3% of these grasp patterns being precise (3 jaw chuck or pincer). She did not demonstrate a controlled release of objects. Instead, she dropped the objects unintentionally or used the left hand to remove the object. No transfers from hand to hand were performed in this pretreatment session.

The operational definitions in Table 6 define for the reader what variables the clinicians observed and characterized. The ICCs (intraclass correlation coefficients) in the far right column of the table give estimates of the interrater reliabilities of the observations. Because the authors provided thorough descriptions of what they did and observed, other therapists can replicate the procedures.

TABLE 6. Criteria for Video Analysis of the Quality and Quantity of Movement

Target UE Behavior	Operational Definition	Attempts per Session (mean)	ICC
Flexor position	Metacarpal phalangeal and proximal interphalangeal joints postured in >90° of flexion	20:57*	0.90
Right reaches[†]	Intentional movement of the involved upper extremity to obtain an object with abduction or flexion of shoulder and/or elbow extension	94.7	0.94
Grasp success	Picking up an object or pellet intentionally and maintaining a grip for at least 1 sec	47.9	0.76
Grasp precision	Use of either a 3-jaw chuck or pincer grasp to obtain an object or pellet	25.6	0.96
Release success	Active finger extension with either a supported or unsupported wrist	14.8	0.96
Release precision	Active finger extension without wrist support	4.6[‡]	0.76
Transfer success[†]	Passing the object from one hand to the other and maintaining a grasp in the receiving hand for >1 sec (body may be used as intermediary)	11.8	0.84
Smooth transfer[†]	Successful transfer with release of the object from one hand and simultaneous grasp with the other hand	10.2[‡]	0.91

*Mean length of total time recorded in minutes.

[†]These measures were analyzed only during periods when the constraint was not on. All other measures were analyzed with and without the constraint.

[‡]Analysis of precision was not possible for all attempts because of camera angle and distance.

UE indicates upper extremity; ICC, intraclass correlation coefficient.

Reprinted with permission of APTA Section on Pediatrics from Fergus A, Buckler J, Farrell J, et al. Constraint-induced movement therapy for a child with hemiparesis: a case report. Pediatr Phys Ther. 2008;20:271-283; Table 1.

TABLE 7. Characteristics of 3 Patients

	Patient 1	Patient 2	Patient 3
Age (y)	60	72	72
Sex	Male	Male	Female
Body mass index (kg/m²)	27.7	25.1	14.1
Baseline UPDRS[a] total score	41	27	17
Baseline Hoehn and Yahr score	2	2	2.5
Premorbid conditions	Arthritis of the right hip	None	Livedo reticularis, bilateral lower extremities
Maximum tolerable treadmill speed (mph)	3.0	2.5	3.5

[a]UPDRAS = Unified Parkinson's Disease Rating Scale

Reprinted from Schenkman M, Hall D, Kumar R, Kohrt WM. Endurance exercise training to improve economy of movement of people with Parkinson disease: three case reports. Phys Ther. 2008;88:63-76; Table 1.

TABLE 8. Impairments in Body Structure and Function as Measured at Baseline

Impairment	Tests and Measures	Finding
Spasticity	Resistance to passive stretch measuring using the modified Ashworth Scale	Right lower extremity: 2 Left lower extremity: 1+
Strength	Manual muscle test (0-5)	4/5 in bilateral lower extremities, except for hip extension and hip abduction bilaterally (3+/5)
Dysmetria	Past pointing Finger to nose Heel to shin	Moderate impairment on all tests
Right heel cord tightness	Goniometry	–2° of neutral
Clonus	Quick stretch	2 beats of clonus on right

Reprinted from Cernak K, Stevens V, Price R, Shumway-Cook A. Locomotor training using body-weight support on a treadmill in conjunction with ongoing physical therapy in a child with severe cerebellar ataxia. Phys Ther. 2008;88:88-97; Table 1.

Depicting Patient Data

Figures and tables can be used to supplement the text and to summarize some of the patient data. Schenkman and colleagues[19] included a table that provided the characteristics of 3 patients in a case report of endurance exercise training in people with Parkinson disease (Table 7). Cernak et al[20] used a table to summarize the impairments in body structures and functions of a child with cerebellar ataxia, the tests and measures used to examine each, and the findings (Table 8).

Alnwick[11] summarized 6 years of a patient's history—a patient with a referral diagnosis of fibromyalgia who actually had serotonin syndrome (Table 9). Cernak et al[20] used a table (Table 10) to show changes in locomotor training parameters and abilities of a child with cerebral ataxia over a 6-month period.

To their case report, Anderson and Tichenor[21] added a figure of the body chart used to identify the anatomical location of the patient's reported pain (Figure 21).

Evaluation

Evaluations are clinical judgments that clinicians make for the purpose of establishing a diagnosis and prognosis. Figure 18 defines these terms as they are used by the *Guide to Physical Therapist Practice*.[2]

Evaluations are based on a synthesis of all of the data that you reported in the systems review and tests-and-measures section. Now it's time to explain your clinical impression and how you used each piece of data to establish a diagnosis, prognosis, and plan of care. Which test results helped rule out a diagnosis? Which data helped you classify the patient's problems? Which results led you toward a diagnosis or classification that you then confirmed with other data? Which pieces of information did you use to arrive at a hypothesis about the cause of the patient's problem? As with every other part of a case report, put your thought process in writing so that it is clear to readers (and to yourself).

Case report writers who clearly describe their evaluation, diagnosis, and prognosis processes make their decision making explicit and contribute valuable examples of these aspects

TABLE 9. Time Line of Events

Time	Event
6 y prior to diagnosis of serotonin syndrome (SS)	The patient began taking citalopram; the exact start date is unknown.
4 y prior to diagnosis of SS	The patient reported intermittent nausea and vomiting with a slow and gradual onset and was considered to have Ménière disease.
2 y prior to diagnosis of SS	Symptoms continued to worsen, with increased bouts of nausea and vomiting daily and increased headaches. The patient consulted numerous specialists, with no significant improvement.
~1 y prior to diagnosis of SS	The patient began to have mental symptoms, such as loss of memory and confusion.
6 mo prior to diagnosis of SS	Symptoms continued to worsen. The patient's short-term memory was worsening, along with an increase in other symptoms and pain.
2 mo prior to diagnosis of SS	The patient was referred for physical therapy for the first time. At this time, the patient was not working, needed assistance with basic activities of daily living (ADL), and was unable to perform instrumental ADL. The patient scored 70% on the first Oswestry Disability Index (ODI) questionnaire.
1 mo prior to diagnosis of SS	The patient scored 62% on the second ODI questionnaire and continued to have many of the same symptoms, but at a slightly lesser degree.
Diagnosis of SS made by neurologist	An initial evaluation was performed by a neurologist. Citalopram was tapered off and discontinued. Within 2 wk of the discontinuation of citalopram, the patient reported significant decreases in all of her symptoms.
3 mo after diagnosis of SS	The patient was discharged from physical therapy and scored 28% on the ODI questionnaire. From referral to discharge from physical therapy, the patient was seen for a total of 41 visits.
9 mo after diagnosis of SS	At a follow-up examination, the patient scored 0% on the ODI questionnaire. She also reported returning to work and hobbies.

Reprinted from Alnwick GM. Misdiagnosis of serotonin syndrome as fibromyalgia and the role of physical therapists. Phys Ther. 2008;88:757-765; Table 1.

of patient/client management by physical therapists. Relatively few such examples exist in the literature. Similarly, few examples of the entire process of evaluation used in making decisions for clients receiving occupational therapy services exist in the literature.

Diagnosis

In the best of all rehabilitation worlds, therapists would be able to identify a cluster (eg, of signs or symptoms, impairments, activity limitations, and participation restrictions), a syndrome, or a category as part of diagnostic classification for all patients, which then would lead to the most appropriate intervention. Unfortunately, this "best of all worlds" does not yet exist—with a few exceptions.

TABLE 10. Parameters for Training on a Treadmill and over ground Training With Body-Weight Support[a]

	Clinical Training (1 mo)				No training (1 mo)	Home Training (4 mo)	
	Week 1 (Pretest)	Week 2	Week 3	Week 4 (Posttest)	1-Month Retention Test	Months 3-4	Months 5-6
Treadmill time (min)	15	15	15	15	15	15	15
Treadmill speed (m/s)	0.18	0.31	0.31	0.31	0.36	0.54	0.54
Body-weight support	30%	25%	20%	15%	15%	10%	10%
No. of rest breaksrequired	2	1	0	0	0	0	0
Amount of assistance	3 people	3 people	3 people	1–3 people	1 person	1 person	CG/SBA
Overground walking time with BWS (min)	5	12	15	15	15	N/A	N/A
Distance walked overground with BWS (m)	50	91	125	157	188	N/A	N/A
Distance with walked overground without BWS (m)						8 with 4WW	152 with U-Step[b]

[a] BWS=body-weight support, N/A=not applicable, CG/SBA=contact guard or standby assist, 4WW=4-wheeled walker.

[b] In-Step Mobility Products Corp, 8027 N Monticello Ave, Skokie, IL 60076.

Reprinted from Cernak K, Stevens V, Price R, Shumway-Cook A. Locomotor training using body-weight support on a treadmill in conjunction with ongoing physical therapy in a child with severe cerebellar ataxia. Phys Ther. 2008;88:88-97; Table 2.

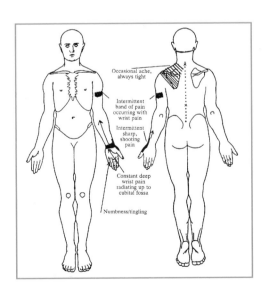

FIGURE 21. Body chart illustrating where the patient reported pain when first examined.

Reprinted from Anderson M, Tichenor CJ. A patient with de Quervain's tenosynovitis: a case report using an Australian approach to manual therapy. *Phys Ther.* 1994;74:314-326.

Classification	Key Signs and Symptoms	Treatment Approach
Extension	Flexion activities worsened symptoms (sitting, bending)	Extension exercises
	Symptoms improved with extension movement testing	Restriction of flexion (education/ bracing)
	Symptoms worsened with flexion movement testing	
Flexion	Extension activities worsened symptoms (standing, walking)	Flexion exercises
	Symptoms improved with flexion movement testing	Restriction of extension (education/bracing)
	Symptoms worsened with extension movement testing	Partially unloaded walking
Mobilization (lumbar/sacroiliac)	Sacroiliac: positive sacroiliac tests	Mobilization/manipulation
	Lumbar: opening or closing pattern with movement testing	
Immobilization	Frequent prior episodes due to minimal spinal perturbations	Avoidance of end-range or sustained postures (bracing/education)
	Prolonged static postures worsened symptoms	Trunk strengthening and stabilization exercises
	Symptoms worsened with sustained movement testing	
	Symptoms improved with repeated movement testing	
Lateral shift	Visible lateral shift (lateral translation of the trunk relative to the pelvis)	Pelvic translocation exercise in standing or prone position
	Asymmetrical side-bending range of motion	Pelvic translocation exercise combined with extension
	Symptoms improved with pelvic translocation movement testing, worsened with opposite translocation	Autotraction
Traction	Radicular symptoms	Mechanical traction
	Symptoms did not improve with any movement tests	Autotraction
	Symptoms worsened with most movement tests	

The *Guide to Physical Therapist Practice* contains preferred practice patterns, into which patients are classified based on the physical therapist's evaluation of the examination data; however, the practice patterns provide only the "boundaries within which a physical therapist may design and implement plans of care."[2(p35)] Case report writers might specify the practice pattern into which they classify the patient, as delineated in the Guide, but they also should provide a more specific diagnosis, if one can be determined. A case report by Fritz[22] gives a good example of a diagnostic classification approach for patients with low back syndrome that is specific and guides intervention (Table 11).

Sometimes the evaluation and the diagnostic process reveal findings that are outside the scope of the therapist's knowledge, experience, or expertise and that therefore require the therapist to refer the patient to an appropriate practitioner.[2] Gray's case report[23] is an example of such a situation. His evaluation indicated that a patient with a referral diagnosis of sciatica might actually have intermittent vascular claudication. The therapist referred the patient back to the physician to rule out occlusive vascular disease, which a vascular specialist subsequently diagnosed and surgically repaired.

When the diagnostic process does not yield an identifiable cluster, syndrome, or category, therapists must develop hypotheses about the cause of the patient's problem and must design possible solutions. The hypothesis may relate to the identification of a particular pathology that the clinician believes to be responsible for the problem, or it may relate to the determination of the impairments that appear to contribute to the activity limitations or the participation restrictions that the patient or someone else, such as a family member, report. In either case, hypothesized causes are critical aspects of clinical decision making. Because the hypothesized causes of the problem link the evaluation to the prognosis and plan of care, authors of case reports are obligated to explain their hypotheses and how the data contributed to them.

In experimental studies, a hypothesis is a *testable* idea about cause. Because case reports lack the controls of experimental studies, hypotheses cannot be tested in the same way they are tested in research. But hypotheses are tested informally in case reports (and in day-to-day practice!) through the data collected and the logical arguments that the author provides.

In *PTJ* case reports, a clinical impression would be included after the diagnosis section that would either confirm the original hypotheses or state new or revised hypotheses based on the examination findings and that would provide the rationale for the treatment approach to be used.

Riddle et al[24(pp479-80)] described a 47-year-old woman with low back pain who was referred for physical therapy. After completing their examination, the authors hypothesized that:

In our opinion, the patient in this case report was unable to achieve her goals because of localized chronic inflammatory processes in the area of the lower 3 vertebrae of the lumbar spine. We also hypothesized that this was a chronic inflammation that appeared to have been precipitated by several impairments. The limited lumbar sagittal-plane motion and lumbar accessory motion appeared to be long-standing and may have predisposed the patient to developing inflammation in the area of the lumbar spine. Because most of the patient's complaints were associated with a flexed lumbar spine, the painful and limited forward ending appeared to be the most important of the 3 impairments associated with movement of the lumbar spine.

Here, the authors *informally* tested their hypothesis by applying an intervention designed to address the factors identified in their hypothesis. Although the patient improved, she did not meet all of her goals. The authors argued that the hypotheses and interventions were appropriate, however, and that if the patient continued the exercise program at home, her morning pain would be eliminated. The patient's outcomes did support the credibility of the hypothesis—but lacking the controls of research, the case report could not prove that the intervention caused the improvements in the patient's condition.

Moyers and Stoffel[25(p641)] proposed and tested a hypothesis regarding a patient scheduled for surgery for recurrent bilateral carpal tunnel syndrome, carpo-metacarpal arthritis of the right thumb, and an osteophyte on the left trapezoid. The examination interview with the patient and her husband suggested that the patient drank an excessive amount of alcohol.

Obviously, continued drinking during treatment could limit the options for controlling postsurgical pain (eg, transcutaneous nerve stimulation in place of medication) (Acute Pain Management Guideline, 1992), could ultimately interfere with the client's progress toward the goals of rehabilitation, could prevent implementation of the second surgical procedure, and could potentially increase the time off from work.

The authors tested their hypothesis by using a motivational interviewing approach, which led to a diagnosis of substance dependence and ultimately to the patient's participation in a detoxification program.

A hypothesis was developed and informally tested by Mossberg et al[13(p81)] with 2 patients with reduced cardiovascular fitness following traumatic brain injury. The authors summarized their findings and then explained their hypothesis:

Results of aerobic testing indicated that both patients were well below the 10th percentile for peak $\dot{V}o_2$ in age- and sex-matched individuals without impairments.[22,23] This finding was not surprising given their respective histories and gait impairments. Moderate to severe balance deficiencies were apparent from the Berg Balance Scale scores. Slow gait speeds and decreased endurance were evident from the results of the 6MW. Both patients complained of fatigue toward the end of the test, and patient 2's safety became compromised. This was accompanied by verbal expressions of frustration and intolerance for the activity.

These findings led to the conclusion that BWSTT would be an appropriate intervention to improve endurance, cardiorespiratory capacity, and the ability to walk unsupported over ground. The body-weight support accommodated the weakness and balance impairments. In addition, it allowed staff to concentrate on gait quality rather than body-weight support. The treadmill provided the higher frequency of stepping and consequently could improve endurance and cardiorespiratory capacity, provided the stimulus was the proper intensity.

When the diagnostic process does not yield an identifiable cluster, syndrome, or category, therapists must develop hypotheses about the cause of the patient's problem and must design possible solutions.

The authors' hypothesis was supported when the patients' cardiorespiratory capacity improved after receiving body weight-supported treadmill training (BWSTT). Because the case report did not have the controls of research, however, they could not claim that BWSTT caused the improvement.

Gill-Body and colleagues[26(p133)] reported on the cases of 2 patients with peripheral vestibular dysfunction, one of whom complained of a 3-month history of difficulty walking outdoors, ringing in the right ear, and an inability to return to work as a tour guide due to her inability to stand on a moving bus and walk in a straight line while maintaining balance. After the examination, the authors hypothesized the following:

1. The patient's decreased cervical range of motion could be related to her voluntarily holding her head still during gait and other functional activities; decreased cervical range of motion and alignment could impair postural responses10 and were therefore worth addressing in intervention.

2. The patient's primary problem of impaired postural stability was related to her vestibular hypofunction on the right side, as supported by the posturography test results of difficulty with sensory conditions 5 and 6 [results obtained with an instrument designed to measure body sway under different conditions].

3. The patient clearly demonstrated some ability to utilize vestibular information for postural control in situations in which accurate visual and proprioceptive information were not as available (ie, sensory conditions 5 and 6 could be partially performed on some trials).

These 3 hypotheses were developed to guide intervention based on the examination findings. The authors devised an intervention program designed to address the impaired balance and range of motion that were identified in the hypotheses. Follow-up balance and range-of-motion measurements were reported after a course of intervention, as were other outcomes. (See **Chapter 8**, "Describing the Outcomes.") The authors provided data to support their hypotheses in the following way: They thoroughly described their intervention and how it was linked to their hypotheses, reported the preintervention and postintervention impairment measurements that were referred to in the hypotheses, and thoroughly described the changes that took place in the patient's functional ability.

Malouin and colleagues[27] took a different approach to informal hypothesis testing. They referenced several studies that supported the hypothesis that intensive and early task-specific training was the rehabilitation approach of choice for patients with acute cerebrovascular accidents who had altered gait patterns. The authors also wanted to thoroughly describe the proposed intervention procedures. They reported a large amount of data to support their conclusion: "Early and intensive gait-related training is feasible and...can be very well tolerated by patients who are moderately to severely involved following a stroke."[27(p788)]

> Justify the pursuit of large, controlled experimental studies

Because they were not conducting a research study, the authors did not test the hypothesis of whether their intervention approach was more effective than another approach. But their report suggested that a true experimental study would be an appropriate next step. This is an example of the role that case reports can play in providing data that can be used to justify large, controlled experimental studies.

Tables and figures can be used to supplement the text describing hypotheses. Vaughn[28] used a table (Table 12) to summarize potential sources of his patient's knee pain and referred pain in the hip and lumbar spine along with the examination findings that ruled out those sources. After ruling out those sources, the author hypothesized[28(pp619-620)]:

The sacroiliac joint mobility tests, as well as the boney landmark positional findings described above, combined with the limited number of local findings at the patient's painful knee, led the examiner to a working diagnosis of sacroiliac joint dysfunction. The author believed that the knee pain was referred from, or at least related to, the sacroiliac joint dysfunction or its associated impairments. There is essentially no literature to support the validity of the tests that led to this clinical impression. However, because the proposed mechanism (lunge exercise) for the SIJ impairment was consistent with the palpatory and mobility findings, the author proceeded with this working diagnosis.

TABLE 12. Summary of the Differential Diagnostic Considerations for the Patient's Knee Pain and the Rationales for Their Elimination as Primary Contributors to the Presentation

Potential Pain Sources at Knee	Rationale for Diagnostic Exclusion
Patellar tracking	Q-angle WNL
Patellar instability	No history of subluxation or locking
Quadriceps and patellar tendinopathy	Location of pain
Pathological plica	No patellar stuttering; location of pain; no fibrotic thickening
Meniscal lesions	No locking, buckling; history did not support with MOI
Bursitis	Location of pain; no swelling
Stress fractures	No abrupt change in training regimen
Osteoarthritis	Age of patient
ITB friction syndrome	Location of pain
Popliteal tenosynovitis	Location of pain
Ligamentous instability	Stress tests were negative

Possible Sources of Referred Pain	Rationale for Diagnostic Exclusion
Hip	Negative special tests, normal ROM
Lumbar spine discogenic	Negative SLR, excellent ROM
Lumbar spine nondiscogenic	Negative spring tests, excellent ROM

Abbreviations: ITB, iliotibial band; MOI, mechanism of injury; ROM, range of motion; SLR, straight leg raise; WNL, within normal limits.

Reproduced from Vaughn DW. Isolated knee pain: a case report highlighting regional interdependence. J Orthop Sports Phys Ther. 2008;38:616-623, Table 2, with permission of the Orthopaedic and Sports Physical Therapy Sections of the American Physical Therapy Association.

Following one session of manual therapy directed to the pubic symphysis and the sacroiliac joint, the patient was able to run without pain in her knee. This outcome supported the author's hypothesis.

Case reports can be designed to informally test a variety of different forms of hypotheses. If you plan to informally test a hypothesis in your case report, ask yourself the following questions: Is the hypothesis stated clearly in the report? Is the theoretical basis for the hypothesis described? Do the data provided in the report support or refute the hypothesis?

Prognosis

Another key feature of a case report is the statement about the patient's prognosis. Derived from the ancient Greek word for "predict," a prognosis is the clinician's judgment about the patient's likely status at some point in the future or about the rate of change in that status over time.[29,30] Using prognostic information, the clinician can describe the natural history of the condition and the degree to which various interventions might influence it. This, in turn, allows the clinician to make an informed decision regarding the goals, and expected outcomes of treatment.

As a case report writer—and as a clinician—how did you decide that a child with cerebral palsy probably will not walk well enough to do what she wants and needs to do and therefore should have a power wheelchair? What did you consider before deciding, for the patient in your case report, that you could reduce the usual time that patients with low back pain receive workers' compensation? How did you decide that a patient with a stroke should be able to use his arm functionally within 2 months? What information made you think that 3 weeks of intervention would help a woman with hypermobility syndrome participate in her favorite recreational activities again?

Establishing an accurate prognosis is a central component of patient management and is of great importance to all stakeholders, including the patient, family members, employers, payers, and other caregivers. As a prediction of future events, a prognosis relies on the clinician's most informed "guess,"[30,31] so it will always have a degree of uncertainty.

The process of determining a prognosis can be straightforward for some patients but quite challenging for others. In many cases, particularly for patients with musculoskeletal problems, the prognosis is strongly influenced by the magnitude of tissue injury combined with the patient's biological capacity for healing these tissues. For example, the time period for most patients to have symptom-reduction following acute lateral ankle sprain is well described,[33] which means that a clinician usually can predict the time course of functional recovery for these patients quite accurately. For some patients, however, a prognosis also can be greatly influenced by other factors, such as medical and psychosocial comorbidities (Figure 22). If a patient with an acute lateral ankle sprain also has peripheral neuropathy, severe vascular disease, and clinical depression, an accurate prognosis would be much more difficult to determine.

To generate a clinically meaningful prognostic statement, consider the outcome of interest and the specific time in the future when it is likely to occur.[29,31] Many published studies provide information that can be used in making a prognosis. For instance, Kennedy and colleagues[33] investigated the rate of functional change in patients undergoing total knee arthroplasty (TKA). Using the Lower Extremity Functional Scale (LEFS)[34] as an outcome of interest, they applied their findings to develop a prognosis at the level of an individual patient. The results from the study suggested that 8 weeks after surgery, a typical patient undergoing TKA probably would have: 1) moderate difficulty performing heavy activities around the house, 2) minimal difficulty ascending and descending stairs, and 3) no difficulty sitting for an hour or walking short distances.

Another example is a study that generated growth curves to predict the rate and limits of gross motor development of children of cerebral palsy.[35] The researchers classified the children using the 5-level Gross Motor Function Classification System (GMFCS)[36] and measured gross motor development over time using the Gross Motor Function Measure.[37] Based on the findings, on average, children classified at level I, with the least severe motor impairments, are predicted to be able to walk down stairs alternating steps without holding a railing by about 5 years of age and to reach their maximum level of gross motor development by about 9 years of age. On average, children classified at level IV, with more severe motor impairments, are predicted to be able to sit unsupported for several seconds by 2 years of age, to reach maximum level of gross motor function by about 5 years, and to never be able to take steps and walk without support. Using the predicted rate and level of development of children classified at these and other GMFCS levels, clinicians can focus intervention on the skills that children are likely to be able to achieve and can predict when compensation—such as through the use of assistive technology—is likely to be necessary for a child to participate. (A caution: this study showed only the predicted development of basic gross motor skills, not functional skills that a child might be able to achieve in spite of gross motor limitations.)

The usefulness of the prognostic statement in a case report can be enhanced by including an estimate of the probability of achieving the outcome of interest.[38,39] Because case reports often

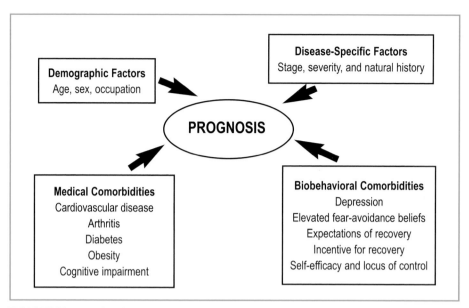

FIGURE 22. Examples of patient characteristics that should be considered when determining a patient's prognosis for outcome following physical therapy intervention.

Reprinted from Beattie PF, Nelson RM. Evaluating research studies that address prognosis for patients receiving physical therapy care. *Phys Ther.* 2007;87:1527-1535; Figure.

describe uncommon patient presentations, little might be known about the specific course of the illness or likely response to treatment, thus the probability estimate often is based on the previous experience and intuition of the clinician. For example, a clinician might predict "a 75% probability that the patient will be able to ambulate 100 meters without assistive device at 1 month following surgery."

Research findings might be available to help you determine the probability of achieving a specific outcome.[30,38-40] Prognostic factors are unique characteristics of patients that research has shown to predict an outcome. These factors are present following the onset of a condition or illness, and they influence (but don't necessarily cause) patient outcomes.[30] Research studies that address prognostic factors measure various patient characteristics at the time of diagnosis or start of care and then statistically determine the degree to which these characteristics are associated with the outcome that the researchers are interested in.[30,39] The "statistical indices" that are derived from these types of studies might, under the right circumstances, be applied to individual patients, allowing the clinician to increase prognostic accuracy by identifying the presence or absence of one or more prognostic factors.

Alphabet Soup: ORs, RRs, LR, and CPRs Help Make Prognoses

Several "statistical indices" have been used to describe the association between an outcome and the presence or absence of a prognostic factor. Indices greater than 1 typically represent an increased probability of a specific outcome, whereas indices less than 1 suggest a reduced probability.

Odds ratios (ORs). The ratio of the odds of an outcome occurring in one group of patients who have a specific trait is compared to that of another group who do not have that trait.[41] Hillard et al,[42] for instance, reported that community-living older people who required multiple steps to regain standing balance following lateral perturbation had an OR of 6.2 for a fall in the future compared with those did not have this trait. In other words, for people in this population, the odds of a fall occurring in those who required multiple steps to recover balance was more than 6 times that of those who did not require multiple steps. Requiring multiple steps to regain balance predicts a poor prognosis compared to people who do not require multiple steps.

Relative risk (RR). This calculation is used to determine if the risk of an outcome—such as the development of a disease—is increased or decreased by the presence or absence of a certain trait. Lang and colleagues[42] assessed the association between physical activity and subsequent physical functioning in middle-aged adults. They reported that the incidence of mobility problems for adults with "normal weight" who were active on 3 or more days per week had an RR of .56 when compared with those who were not active 3 or more days per week; that is, those who were frequently active had a much lower risk of subsequent mobility problems.

Likelihood ratio (LR). The LR is calculated using the sensitivity and specificity of a given prognostic factor's capacity to determine an outcome of interest.[44] Riddle and Stratford[45] reported that patients with a Berg Balance Scale (BBS) score of <40 had a positive LR of 11.7; that is, on average, patients with scores of 40 or less on the BBS were nearly 12 times more likely to fall than patients who scored over 40. Likelihood ratios are valuable because they can be used to assess the strength of a prognostic factor to influence outcome after considering the pretest likelihood of that outcome.

How does prediction work in practice? The clinician uses past experience and knowledge to judge the pretest probability of a specific outcome occurring, based on medical history and other physical examination findings, and then applies the LRs to determine how much a certain test result increases or decreases the probability of that outcome. Using the data described by Riddle and Stratford,[45] 2 patients might both have a BBS score of <40; however, one patient might have medical comorbidities that increase the likelihood of falling compared with the other.

Let's look at 2 hypothetical patients to illustrate this example. Patient #1 is found to have relatively serious medical comorbidities that—experience and published evidence suggest—increase the patient's risk for falls. The physical therapist, therefore, might estimate that the risk for falls in Patient #1 is 50%. For Patient #2, no comorbidities were identified, so the therapist might estimate that the pretest probability for falls in Patient #2 is low—say, only 5%. Using the nomogram in Figure 23, the therapist finds that, after obtaining the BBS score for Patient #1, the patient's risk for falls increases to approximately 90%. For Patient #2 (the one with a pretest probability of falls of only 5%), the posttest probability after obtaining the BBS score also increases, but to only about 40%. This type of information may be extremely helpful to the therapist in determining appropriate interventions, given the differing risks of falls for the 2 patients.

       Clinical prediction rules (CPRs). Clinical prediction rules that address prognosis may be derived from longitudinal studies by statistically combining multiple prognostic factors to yield a single measure of statistical likelihood of an outcome of interest.[46] A great advantage of CPRs is that they can be very helpful in developing a quantitative prognostic statement when considering many patient characteristics. Lesher and colleagues[47] reported that the presence of a positive patellar tilt test and tibia varum of greater than 5 degrees increased the likelihood of an immediate successful response to patellar taping from 52% to 83%. Although the presence of these 2 findings is likely to improve the prognosis of patients with patellofemoral pain syndrome who are receiving patellar taping, clinicians need to make sure that a CPR has adequate validation to be applied to their own individual patients. In other words, the patients and techniques used by the researchers must be similar to the patient and environment in which the rule will be applied.[46]

FIGURE 23. A nomogram illustrating how a patient's comorbidities increase the likelihood of falling compared with another patient.

Adapted from Riddle DL, Stratford PW. Interpreting validity indexes for diagnostic tests: an illustration using the Berg Balance Test. *Phys Ther.* 1999;79:939-948.

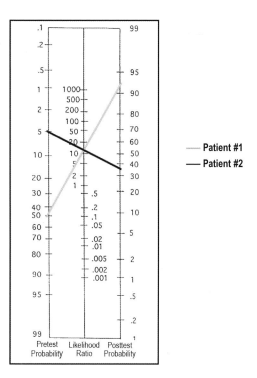

Patient #1

Patient #2

What If There's No Research to Help With Prognosis?

More and more research is becoming available to help rehabilitation professionals determine a prognosis; however, if you can't find research, you probably can make a presumptive argument for the prognosis. **Chapter 4** described how to make a presumptive argument for the reliability and validity of measurements; making a presumptive argument to support your prognosis is similar. The clinician develops theoretical arguments to support the decisions involved in determining a prognosis. Even if you cannot find research reports, perhaps your literature search will reveal clinical perspectives, case reports, and other peer-reviewed observations and opinions about the prognosis for patients who are similar to yours. Perhaps you can find related research that addresses certain aspects of the patient's problem—such as the healing time for soft tissue injuries—from which you can make a presumptive argument about the prognosis for a patient's specific type of injury.

Sometimes clinicians have no alternative other than to base the prognosis on their own past experience or the experience of colleagues. If you base the prognosis on experience, make sure that you clearly state whose experience it was. Too many authors use the passive voice to avoid using the first person. An example: "It has been observed that most patients with these examination results are independent in ADL within 2 months." Who made this observation? The passive voice ("it has been observed") hides the actor. A clearer statement would be: "I have observed that most patients…."

Except in rare instances, avoid determining a prognosis based solely on your own experience. In a case report of a patient with hypermobility syndrome (HMS), Russek[48(p392)] used a combination of published opinion, a presumptive argument, and her own experience to determine a prognosis:

> Avoid a prognosis based solely on your own experience

> Prognosis for HMS is mixed. On one hand, there is no cure for the disorder. The goal for treatment, therefore is not to return to "normal" (ie, not hypermobile) joint mobility but restoration of relatively pain-free function. That is, treatment does not eliminate the underlying impairment of excessive mobility. However, physicians specializing in HMS propose that treatment improves function and decreases disability.[6,35]

> Some authors[2,12,36-39] assert that HMS is not progressive and does not necessarily lead to progressive deformity or disability in the way that rheumatoid arthritis, for example, might. From this point of view, the prognosis is good. Individuals with HMS, however, have a greater incidence of many acute and chronic musculoskeletal disorders[5,11] and tend to develop more osteoarthritis than individuals without hypermobility.[3,40,41] Hypermobility syndrome also is associated with some other systemic disorders, such as mitral valve prolapse.[6] Overall, therefore, prognosis is fair to good. In the opinion of some physicians and my clinical experience, patients with HMS can function and their quality of life often can be improved with treatment but they will usually have chronic or recurrent problems.

Note that Russek did not include a time line for improvement. Today, reviewers, editors, and most instructors expect to see that kind of time line.

Patient Description Guideposts

■ Why did the patient receive physical therapy? Only the relevant details of the history of the problem should be included in the case report. The complete prenatal and birth history of a person with cerebral palsy, for instance, usually isn't necessary; note only the reason for the current episode of physical therapy. Do include the physician's diagnosis of the problem (if any) and any other diagnoses or history that could influence the course of physical therapy or the outcomes. Current medication, previous surgical/ medical history, and prior physical therapy for other problems are examples of information that could be important in understanding your case.

■ What contextual factors, such as patient behaviors and social and environmental factors, may have affected physical therapy and outcomes? Physical therapists are acutely aware of the importance of psychological, social, and environmental factors and their impact on patient outcomes. Although it is beyond physical therapists' scope of practice to diagnose psychological or social problems, we can describe patient behaviors and personal, social, and environmental factors that may affect physical therapy and outcomes. A supportive family, the desire to go back to school, a home with architectural barriers—these are just a few examples of the countless factors that enter into the clinical decision-making process and have a critical influence on outcomes.

■ Did the patient receive other services? Physical therapy may not be the only intervention that patients receive, particularly if the problem is long-standing or if the patient has multiple problems. A patient with neck pain, for instance, may have seen other health care professionals before arriving in your clinic. A patient with a stroke could be receiving occupational therapy, speech-language pathology services, rehabilitation nursing, and therapeutic recreation services. Although case reports cannot sort out the relative contribution of physical therapy and other services to outcomes, case reports should describe the other services in relation to the comprehensiveness of patient care.

■ Were there any other problems that could have influenced the anticipated goals and expected outcomes and the means to achieve them? Was the patient grossly overweight? Did the patient have seizures? Did the patient have a serious cognitive deficit? These and other comorbidities could influence the course of physical therapy interventions and outcomes.

■ How well did the patient understand the problem? The patient's understanding can influence physical therapy and outcomes. In general, patients who have a good understanding of the problem are more likely to have better outcomes than those who do not.

■ What did the patient want to accomplish? The *Guide to Physical Therapist Practice*[1] and APTA's "Guidelines for Physical Therapy Documentation"[2] emphasize that patients/clients and their significant others should participate in establishing the anticipated goals and expected goals and that these goals and outcomes should be "stated in measurable terms." The goals of both the patient and the people who are important in the patient's life must drive the physical therapy plan of care. Functional outcomes can usually be identified by listening to what the patient wants to be able to do, such as, "I want to be able to work all day," "I want to play in the first game of the season," or "I want to be able to walk to the bathroom by myself." Measurement of the level of achievement of goals should be included in case reports.

References

1 Guide to Physical Therapist Practice. 2nd ed. Phys Ther. 2001;81:9-744. Revised June 2003.

2 Guidelines: Physical Therapy Documentation of Patient/Client Management. BOD G03-05-16-41. American Physical Therapy Association Web site. http://www.apta.org/AM/Template.cfm?Section=Policies_and_Bylaws&TEMPLATE= /CM/ContentDisplay. cfm&CONTENTID=31688. Accessed January 21, 2009.

Plan of Care

According to the *Guide to Physical Therapist Practice*,[2(p46)] the plan of care includes "the anticipated goals and expected outcomes, predicted level of optimal improvement, specific interventions to be used, and proposed duration and frequency of the interventions that are required to reach the anticipated goals and expected outcomes." The *Occupational Therapy Practice Framework*[4] also describes elements for an intervention plan: objective and measurable goals with a time frame; intervention approach based on theory and evidence and mechanisms for service delivery; discharge needs and plan; outcome measures; and recommendations or referral to others as needed.

Mastos et al[49] described a specific goal for a woman with severe traumatic brain injury who wanted to be able to put her hair in a pony tail. They scaled the goals using goal attainment scaling to allow for more precise evaluation of outcomes than a single goal would allow (Table 13).

If you look at case reports published to date, you will find that the authors almost always described the elements of the plan of care or the intervention plan, but they rarely described the decision making that led to each element. Reviewers, editors, and instructors look for descriptions of how case report writers made their decisions. As you write your case report, be sure you answer the question "why" as it relates to each element of the plan. Why these goals? Why this intervention to achieve the goals? Why this amount, frequency, and duration of intervention? As with other parts of your case report, make your decision making explicit! A good way to make all of this explicit is to include it in another statement of a clinical impression that summarizes the working diagnosis, prognosis, plan of care, plan for measurement of outcomes and any other testing, and states why the patient continues to be appropriate for the purpose of the case.

TABLE 13. Goal Selection and Scaling for Case Study 2: Lynn

Goal Attainment Scale: Tying a ponytail		
Attainment level	**Score**	**Securing hair up in a ponytail with a hairband**
Baseline	-2	Lynn gathers hair with her (R) hand, stabilizes hair with (L) hand while hairband is brought once around the gathered hair with her (R) hand.
Less than expected outcome	-1	Above activity+able to insert fingers and thumb of (L) hand inside hairband.
Expected outcome	0	Above activity+able to twist hairband and secure a quarter of her hair with the second loop of the hairband.
Greater than expected outcome	+1	Lynn is able to secure 90% of her hair in a ponytail with the second loop of the hairband.
Much greater than expected outcome	+2	Lynn is able to securely place her hair up in a ponytail using a variety of hairbands.

Mastos M, Miller K, Eliasson AC, Imms C. Clinical Rehabilitation. 2007;21(1):47-55. © 2007 by SAGE Publications. Reprinted by permission of SAGE.

Next: What Did You Do, and Why and How Did You Do It?

Describing your patient or situation and the decision-making process leading to the intervention (if any) involves clarifying your clinical reasoning for the reader. Your rationale for the intervention that you used should be closely linked to the diagnosis or the hypothesized cause of the patient's problem and to the prognosis.

References

1 DeBakey L, DeBakey S. The case report, I: guidelines for preparation. *Int J Cardiol.* 1983;4:357-364.

2 Guide to Physical Therapist Practice. 2nd ed. *Phys Ther.* 2001;81:9-746.

3 Moyers PA, Dale LM. *The Guide to Occupational Therapy Practice.* 2nd ed. Bethesda, MD: American Occupational Therapy Association; 2007.

4 Occupational therapy practice framework: domain and process, ed 2. *Am J Occup Ther.* 2008;62:625–683.

5 Squires BP. Case reports: what editors want from authors and peer reviewers. *Can Med Assoc J.* 1989;141:379-380.

6 Crow JB, Gelfand B, Su EP. Use of joint mobilization in a patient with severely restricted hip motion following bilateral hip resurfacing arthroplasty. *Phys Ther.* 2008;88:1591-1600.

7 Bellamy SG, Gibbs K, Lazaro R. Physical therapy intervention for an adolescent with a knee flexion contracture and diagnosis of multiple pterygium syndrome. *Pediatr Phys Ther.* 2007;19:140-147.

8 Dunbar SB. A child's occupational performance: considerations of sensory processing and family context. *Am J Occup Ther.* 1999;53:231-235.

9 Ellenbecker TS, Bailie DS, Lamprecht D. Humeral resurfacing hemiarthroplasty with meniscal allograft in a young patient with glenohumeral osteoarthritis. *J Orthop Sports Phys Ther.* 2008;38:277-286.

10 Vaughn HT, Nitsch W. Ilial anterior rotation hypermobility in a female collegiate tennis player. *Phys Ther.* 2008;88:1578-1590.

11 Alnwick GM. Misdiagnosis of serotonin syndrome as fibromyalgia and the role of physical therapists. *Phys Ther.* 2008;88:757-765.

12 Fitzgerald GK. Focus and value added: the new case report. *Phys Ther.* 2007;87:494-495.

13 Mossberg KA, Orlander E, Norcross JL. Cardiorespiratory capacity after weight-supported treadmill training in patients with traumatic brain injury. *Phys Ther.* 2008;88:77-87.

14 Chatham K, Gelder CM, Lines TA, Cahalin LP. Suspected statin-induced respiratory muscle myopathy during long-term inspiratory muscle training in a patient with diaphragmatic paralysis. *Phys Ther.* 2009;89:3: 257-266.

15 Elstein AS, Shulman L, Sprafka S. Medical problem solving: a ten-year retrospective. *Eval Health Prof.* 1990;13:5-36.

16 Payton OD. Clinical reasoning process in physical therapy. *Phys Ther.* 1985;65:924-928.

17 Beattie P. The use of an eclectic approach for the treatment of low back pain: a case study. *Phys Ther.* 1992;72:923-928.

18 Fergus A, Buckler J, Farrell J, et al., Constraint-induced movement therapy for a child with hemiparesis: a case report. *Pediatr Phys Ther.* 2008;20:271-283.

19 Schenkman M, Hall D, Kumar R, Kohrt WM. Endurance exercise training to improve economy of movement of people with Parkinson disease: three case reports. *Phys Ther.* 2008;88:63-76.

20 Cernak K, Stevens V, Price R, Shumway-Cook A. Locomotor training using body-weight support on a treadmill in conjunction with ongoing physical therapy in a child with severe cerebellar ataxia. *Phys Ther.* 2008;88:88-97.

21 Anderson M, Tichenor CJ. A patient with de Quervain's tenosynovitis: a case report using an Australian approach to manual therapy. *Phys Ther.* 1994;74:314-326.

22 Fritz JM. Use of a classification approach to the treatment of 3 patients with low back syndrome. *Phys Ther.* 1998;78:766-777.

23 Gray JC. Diagnosis of intermittent vascular claudication in a patient with a diagnosis of sciatica. *Phys Ther.* 1999;79:582-590.

24 Riddle DL, Rothstein JM, Echternach JL. Application of the HOAC II: an episode of care for a patient with low back pain. *Phys Ther.* 2003;83:471-485.

25 Moyers PA, Stoffel VC. Alcohol dependence in a client with a work-related injury. *Am J Occup Ther.* 1999;53:640-645.

26 Gill-Body K, Krebs DE, Parker SW, Riley PO. Physical therapy management of peripheral vestibular dysfunction: two clinical case reports. *Phys Ther.* 1994;74:129-142.

27 Malouin F, Potvin M, Prévost J, et al. Use of an intensive task-oriented gait training program in a series of patients with acute cerebrovascular accidents. *Phys Ther.* 1992;72:781-793.

28 Vaughn DW. Isolated knee pain: a case report highlighting regional interdependence. *J Orthop Sports Phys Ther.* 2008;38:616-623.

29 Straus SE, Richardson WS, Glasziou P, et al. Prognosis. In: *Evidence-Based Medicine.* 3rd ed. New York, NY: Elsevier-Churchill-Livingstone; 2005:101-114.

30 Beattie PF, Nelson RM. Evaluating Research Studies That Address Prognosis for Patients Receiving Physical Therapy Care. *Phys Ther.* 2007;87:1527-1535.

31 Sackett DL, Haynes RB, Tugwell P. Making a prognosis. In: *Clinical Epidemiology: A Basic Science for Clinical Medicine.* Boston, MA: Little, Brown and Company; 1985:159-170.

32 Aiken AB, Pelland L, Brison R, et al. Short-term natural recovery of ankle sprains following discharge from emergency departments. *J Orthop Sports Phys Ther.* 2008;38:566-571.

33 Kennedy DW, Stratford PW, Riddle DL, et al. Assessing recovery and establishing prognosis following total knee arthroplasty. *Phys Ther.* 2008;88:22-32.

34 Binkley JM, Stratford PW, Lott SA, Riddle DL. The Lower Extremity Functional Scale (LEFS): scale development, measurement properties, and clinical application. North American Orthopaedic Rehabilitation Research Network. *Phys Ther.* 1999;79:371-83.

35 Rosenbaum PL, Walter SD, Hanna SE, et al. Prognosis for gross motor function in cerebral palsy: creation of motor development curves. *JAMA.* 2002; 288:1357-1363.

36 Palisano RJ, Rosenbaum PL, Walter SD, Russell DJ, Wood EP, Galuppi BE. Development and reliability of a system to classify gross motor function in children with cerebral palsy. *Dev Med Child Neurol.* 1997;39:214-223.

37 Russell DJ, Rosenbaum PL, Cadman DT, et al. The gross motor function measure. *Dev Med Child Neurol.* 1989;31:341-352.

38 Laupacis A, Wells G, Richardson WS, et al. Users guide to medical literature: V. How to use an article about prognosis. *JAMA.* 1994;272:234-237.

39 De Bie R. Critical appraisal of prognostic studies: An introduction. *Physiotherapy Theory and Practice.* 2001;17:161-172.

40 Hayden J, Bombardier C. Evaluation of the quality of prognosis studies in systematic reviews. *Annals of Internal Medicine.* 2006;144:427-437.

41 Levangie PK Application and interpretation of simple odds ratios in physical therapy-related research. *J Orthop Sports Phys Ther.* 2001;31:496-503.

42 Hillard MJ, Martinez KM, Janssen I, et al. Lateral balance factors predict future falls in community-living older adults. *Arch Phys Med Rehabil.* 2008;89:1708-1713.

43 Lang IA, Gurainik JM, Metzer D. Physical activity in middle-aged adults reduces risk of functional impairment independent of its effect on weight. *Clin J Sport Med.* 2008;18:375-376.

44 Simel DL, Samsa GP, Matchar DB. Likelihood ratios with confidence intervals: sample size estimation for diagnostic test studies. *J Clin Epidemiol.* 1991;44:763-770.

45 Riddle DL, Stratford PW. Interpreting validity indexes for diagnostic tests: an illustration using the Berg Balance Test. *Phys Ther.* 1999;79:939-948.

46 Beattie PF, Nelson RM. Clinical Prediction Rules: What are they and what do they tell us? *Aust J Physiother.* 2006;52:157-163.

47 Lesher JD, Sutlive TG, Miller GA, et al. Development of a clinical prediction rule for classifying patients with patellofemoral pain syndrome who respond to patellar taping. *J of Orthop Sports Phys Ther.* 2006;36:854-866.

48 Russek LN. Examination and treatment of a patient with hypermobility syndrome. *Phys Ther.* 2000:80:386-389.

49 Mastos M, Miller K, Eliasson AC, Imms C. Goal-directed training: linking theories of treatment to clinical practice for improved functional activities in daily life. *Clinical Rehabilitation.* 2007;21(1):47-55.

CHAPTER 8

Describing the Intervention

If case reports are to be useful to clinicians
and are to serve as a basis for experimental studies,
descriptions of the intervention rationale must be
complete and understandable.

Afterdescribing the patient (or other entity), the examination, the evaluation,
diagnosis, and prognosis, the next step is to describe what was done to reach the
identified goals—that is, the next step is to describe the intervention. When the focus
of the case report is an entity other than a patient, the "intervention" can take many forms. Both
the decision-making process that led to the intervention decisions and the components of the
intervention should be clearly described.

What Was Your Rationale for the Intervention?

Unfortunately, many case reports published in the rehabilitation literature do not
adequately describe the rationale that the author used in deciding what interventions to use and
how to apply them. The rationale for intervention is part of the decision-making process
described in **Chapter 6**. Depending on the flow of the case report, the intervention and its
rationale could be addressed under the subhead of "introduction," "prognosis," "plan of care,"[1]
"intervention plan,"[2] or "intervention." In any case, the rationale must be addressed. Today,
editors, reviewers, and instructors make certain that it is!

Clinical decisions related to interventions can be classified into 2 types: those that relate to
the type and amount of intervention initially chosen, and those that relate to why an intervention
approach should be modified. The information reported in a case report to support these 2 types

of decisions can come from a variety of sources, including published research reports, arguments for biological plausibility, and theoretical arguments that have been published in books or journals. You do not always have to reference the work of others when explaining why you made your intervention decisions; however, citing previously published work greatly strengthens the basis of many intervention decisions. Other intervention decisions may be based on the clinical environment or on the patient's environment. "Logic" and "common sense" may serve as a basis for intervention decisions, but the rationale must be consistent with existing evidence about the effectiveness or ineffectiveness of the intervention approach.

The good news is that research evidence is increasingly available to support intervention decisions. There is no universally accepted way to directly apply group data from a study to an individual patient, but many researchers are reporting estimates of the magnitude of a treatment effect—and these estimates can help clinicians interpret research results for application to their own patients.

Calculations You Can Use

Common estimates of treatment effect include relative risk reduction (RRR), absolute risk reduction (ARR), and number needed to treat (NNT), all of which are calculated from dichotomous data[3] (results with 2 categories of outcome, such as the number of patients who improved and didn't improve or the number who went home following total knee arthroplasty and the number who went to an extended care facility). With continuous interval- or ratio-level data, such as degrees of motion, time, and temperature, effect size (ES) can be calculated.[4] That is, authors could calculate and report RRR, ARR, NNT, or ES (we'll spell them out from now on), or a clinician reader could calculate them as long as the research report provides the necessary data.

What does this mean for the writer of a case report? These kinds of calculations, based on published research, could contribute to the rationale for why interventions were selected for a given patient.

Here's how these calculations work in real life:

Just because a study shows that an intervention is effective based on the grouped data of the study participants does not necessarily mean that all of the patients improved. Relative risk reduction and absolute risk reduction are calculations that allow you to interpret the results of a study in terms of your individual patient. The concept of risk is something that rehabilitation clinicians don't usually consider, but risk reduction is becoming "the lingua franca for describing outcomes for therapy."[5(p287)] *Risk* could mean the risk of an intervention being ineffective for a patient or even the risk of an intervention causing an adverse outcome.[5]

Risk of "bad outcomes." Relative risk reduction and absolute risk reduction are based on research that compares the outcomes of intervention and control groups. Relative risk reduction is the proportional reduction in the rates of bad outcomes of patients in the experimental group compared with patients in the control group.[6] It's calculated by subtracting the experimental group's event rate from the control group's event rate and then dividing by the control group's event rate. The event rate is simply the percent of patients who did not improve according to some criterion. As an example, if 12% of patients in the experimental group did not improve and 25% of patients in the control group did not improve, the relative risk reduction would be 52%. In other words, the intervention reduced the risk of a bad outcome by 52% (25% - 12%/25%).

A problem with using relative risk reduction to support an intervention decision is that relative risk reduction does not discriminate between large and small treatment effects.[6] Calculating absolute risk reduction overcomes this problem. Absolute risk reduction is the absolute arithmetic difference in rates of bad outcomes of patients in the experimental and control groups.[6] It's calculated by simply subtracting the experimental group's event rate from the control group's event rate. If 12% of patients in the experimental group did not improve and 25% in the control group did not improve, the absolute risk reduction would be 13%. In other words, the intervention reduced the risk of a bad outcome by 13% (25% - 12%). A clinician would need to decide if a 13% reduction in the risk of a bad outcome is enough to warrant trying the intervention. If so, the author could use the 13% absolute risk reduction to support the decision.

Number needed to treat for one patient to benefit. Another useful way to interpret the magnitude of a treatment effect is the number needed to treat, that is, the number of patients who need to receive the intervention to prevent one additional bad outcome—or, put another way, the number who need to receive the intervention in order for one patient to benefit.[3] The number needed to treat is the inverse of absolute risk reduction; so, using the example above, the inverse of 13% (1/13%) is 8. This means that 8 patients would need to receive an intervention for one to benefit. Depending on such considerations as the consequences of the "bad outcome" and the cost of the intervention, a clinician or patient would have to decide if the intervention is worth trying. Larger magnitude treatment effects are associated with smaller number-needed-to-treat values. A number needed to treat of less than 10 indicates that the experimental treatment was at least 10% better than the comparison treatment or no treatment.

Effect size. Researchers could calculate and report effect size if the outcome data are continuous (eg, distance, time, degrees). If given the necessary information, clinicians can calculate effect sizes themselves. The effect size reflects the magnitude of the observed differences between intervention and comparison or control groups.[7] Guidelines for interpreting effect sizes in behavioral sciences have been provided for small (.20), moderate (.50), and large (.80) effects.[4] Portney and Watkins[7] caution that values are relative and must be operationalized (see **Chapter 4**), saying that what is considered to be a small effect size for tests of movement, for example, may be different from a small effect for psychological measurements. To interpret effect sizes, they suggest that a small effect size is not perceptible to the human eye, a medium effect size is visible to the human eye, and a large effect size clearly shows differences between groups.

To calculate an effect size, the first step is to determine the mean difference in the data of the experimental and comparison or control groups. The second step is to calculate a pooled standard deviation (weighted by sample size) for the groups. The effect size is calculated by dividing the mean difference by the pooled standard deviation.

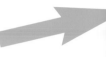

Remember that randomized controlled trials that yield relative risk reduction, absolute risk reduction, number needed to treat, or effect size are not often available for making decisions—and, even if they are available, they can provide justification for only a part of an intervention. As we'll see, case report writers have described many different types of rationales for their interventions.

What Made You Choose the *Initial* Intervention?

One way of explaining rationale for an intervention is found in the case report of Vaughn,[8(p620)] who explained why he chose the initial intervention for a patient with knee pain, which Vaughn hypothesized was caused by sacroiliac dysfunction:

> [I] decided to mobilize the pubic symphysis, first using the method described by Greenman.[17] The rationale for this decision was based on Greenman's[17] and Isaac's[18] contention that pubic symphysis dysfunction should be addressed prior to most dysfunctions in the sacroiliac joint. Undoubtedly, given the ring structure of the pelvis, treatment directed at either articulation will influence the other.

In a case report involving the use of a commercially available gaming console with an adolescent who has cerebral palsy, Deutsch et al[9(p1201)] explained why they chose this intervention:

> The goal of the intervention was to determine the feasibility of introducing this novel gaming technology to address a specific patient's goals. We selected the gaming system based on several factors. First, the handheld interface to the virtual world reads acceleration changes to map the movements of the person into the gaming environment. This type of system encourages movements that can be performed in both sitting and standing positions. The patient was able to learn the movements in a sitting position and then practice them in a standing position. Second, there are stock games available in the system that can be analyzed for their biomechanics and motor control requirements. The games then were selected based on patient interest and task requirements. Third, it provides users with knowledge of performance (KP) and knowledge of results (KR). Knowledge of performance is information about the kinematics of the movement, and knowledge of results is information about the outcome of the movement,[32] which have been shown to improve performance and skill in children with CP.[33,34] Finally, it allowed for multiple users, and we were interested in probing how interaction with other users (in this case, the therapists and a child who was developing typically) would be received by the patient.

Many intervention regimens are designed to increase patients' endurance. In the introduction of their case report, Schenkman et al[10(p64)] described their rationale for an endurance exercise program for people with Parkinson disease (PD):

> Relatively little evidence exists regarding endurance exercise training for people with PD. Yet endurance exercise training can be accomplished at a local health club or at home without equipment (eg, brisk walking) and with relatively little training. Even for people with

A clinician is writing a case report about treatment for a patient with lateral elbow pain and wants to include information on the treatment effect for a manipulation technique used in the case. The clinician finds a randomized trial in which one group received the manipulation technique and a comparison group received ultrasound, transverse friction massage, and stretching and strengthening exercises.[1] The research report provided information on 3- and 6-week outcomes for each group. The primary outcome for the trial was a categorical (dichotomous) measure of global improvement (Table).[1] The event rates (improvement) at 3 weeks were 62% for patients receiving manipulation and 20% for those receiving the comparison treatments. The difference in the event rates (absolute rate reduction) was 42%, resulting in a number needed to treat (NNT) (inverse of the absolute rate reduction) of 2.4. Using the 6-week data to perform the same calculations yields an event rate difference of 18% and an NNT of 5.5

Secondary outcomes for the trial were various continuous measures related to pain, and the clinician is most interested in pain ratings during the day. The mean difference between the treatment groups at 3 weeks was .9, and the pooled standard deviation was approximately 2.1. The resulting effect size was .43. Using the 6-week data to perform the same calculations yields an effect size of .88.

Here is one way, but not the only way, to report this information in a case report. Suggesting that this treatment was effective for the patient described in the case report would be inappropriate; however, this information does provide general support for the clinician's use of wrist manipulation:

> Some randomized trial evidence[1] is available to support the use of the wrist manipulation for the patient in this case report. NNTs were lower than 10 for 3- and 6-week global improvement outcomes for patients receiving the wrist manipulation compared with those receiving ultrasound, transverse friction massage, and stretching and strengthening exercises. Furthermore, when pain intensity was measured during the day, the group that had manipulation had an improvement that corresponded with a large effect size (.43) at 6 weeks.

Reference

1 Struijs PA, Damen PJ, Bakker EW, et al. Manipulation of the wrist for management of lateral epicondylitis: a randomized pilot study. Phys.Ther. 2003;83:608-616.

Outcomes from Randomized Trial of Wrist Manipulation for Elbow Pain[a]

Outcome Measure	After 3 weeks			After 6 weeks		
	Group 1	Group 2	P	Group 1	Group 2	P
Global improvement, no. of subjects (%)	8/13[c] (62%)	3/15[c] (20%)	.05	11/13 (85%)	10/15 (67%)	.40
Subjects' main complaint, mean decrease[b]						
X̄	2.6	2.1	.57	4.4	3.7	.33
SD	1.7	2.2		1.5	2.7	
Pain at the moment, mean decrease[b]						
X̄	1.9	1.5	.34	3.1	2.7	.27
SD	2.7	2.6		2.5	3.4	
Pain during day, mean decrease[b]						
X̄	2.6	1.7	.18	5.2[d]	3.2[d]	.03
SD	2.6	1.6		2.4	2.1	
Inconvenience, mean decrease[b]						
X̄	3.0	2.3	.22	4.8	3.7	.19
SD	3.2	2.7		2.6	2.7	
Pain-free grip force (PFGF), mean increase (kg)						
X̄	5.8	3.7	.11	14.8	8.5	.13
SD	11.1	11.5		17.3	10.6	
Maximum grip force, mean increase (kg)						
X̄	1.8	-0.3	.13	6.2	4.0	.15
SD	10.0	7.4		10.5	11.7	
Ratio PFGF/MGF for noninjured arm, mean increase						
X̄	0.1	0.1	.66	0.3	0.2	.31
SD	0.2	0.2		0.3	0.2	
Pressure pain, mean increase (kg/cm^2)						
X̄	0.7	0.5	.12	1.6	0.7	.18
SD	1.0	0.6		2.0	0.8	
Ratio PP/PP for noninjured arm, mean increase						
X̄	0.2	0.1	.20	0.3	0.3	.55
SD	0.3	0.3		0.2	0.3	

[a]Group 1=subjects who received manipulation of the wrist, group 2=subjects who received ultrasound, friction massage, and muscle stretching and strengthening exercises.

[b]Score on a numeric rating scale of 0 to 10, where 0="no complaints" and 10="very severe complaints."

[c]Significant differences (Fisher exact test, df=1, $\alpha \leq .05$) between groups.

[d]Significant differences (independent t test, df=26).

significant bradykinesia, treadmill training can be used for cardiovascular endurance by increasing the treadmill grade to increase demand of the task. Therefore, it would be useful to understand the potential benefits for people with PD.

Endurance exercise training is of particular interest because of the mounting evidence that people with PD have altered cardiovascular function, compared with their counterparts who are healthy. Although maximal aerobic power in individuals with PD is similar to or only slightly lower than in age- and sex-matched individuals who are healthy, the attainment of peak aerobic power occurs at a significantly lower exercise level (eg, lower speed or grade on a treadmill test) in those with PD, indicating poor metabolic efficiency (ie, increased energy cost of the work performed).[9-11]

Interventions often change over time as patients improve or do not improve. Case report authors need to explain and justify changes in the intervention, just as they explained and justified the initial intervention.

What Made You Decide to *Modify* the Intervention?

Carlson and Hadlock[11(p187)] gave a rationale for the exercise program of a patient with postpolio syndrome following rotator cuff repair and described their criteria for progression of the exercises:

> Exercise was started with PROM, and the patient's sister was taught to administer the PROM at home. Then AROM was initiated at the next visit with no ill effects. At the end of the first week of intervention (6 weeks postoperatively), the patient performed 2 proprioceptive neuromuscular facilitation (PNF) patterns (D1 and D2, 5 repetitions each) actively with no pain until the pattern was correctly executed. The patient learned abbreviated ROM patterns when PNF was first introduced due to ROM and strength limitations.
>
> As the patient progressed, the physical therapist made minor corrections of her performance, and home program adjustments were made to progress the home exercise program. The physical therapist chose PNF patterns because the dynamic incorporation of movement patterns in PNF mimics functional movement much better than isolated muscle actions do and because multiple planar movements can be addressed in each multiplanar pattern. The PNF exercises are believed to stimulate weaker muscles to act by linking them to the stronger muscles participating in the patterned movement.[75] The patient performed 2 sets, 8 repetitions per set, of each movement pattern twice daily. When the patient could perform 12 repetitions each time without pain or fatigue, the resistance (Thera-Band tubing) was increased. Yellow tubing was introduced with the patterns in the clinic with no pain reported by the patient. The PNF patterns with yellow tubing then were added as a daily home program, with instructions to the patient to cease the exercise if she encountered pain.

Flowers et al[12(p65)] devoted a major portion of their case report about a patient with finger extensor tendon lacerations to a description of the progression of intervention based on the reexamination and reevaluation. A small sample of their decision making:

The patient was unable to return to the clinic for 5 days … , at which time a 5-degree improvement in the extension lag (25°) was noted along with no change in flexion (90°). We were encouraged, but reluctant to place too much emphasis on only a 5-degree change in measurement. No change was made in the program.... (7 days later), the extension lag had improved to 20 degrees and the flexion increased back to 90 degrees. The improving extension was interpreted as evidence of desirable remodeling at the attenuated repair site. The persistent 20-degree extension lag, however, also suggested a potential tendon adhesion. It was now approximately 8 weeks postsurgery. A decision was made to institute gentle resistive extension exercise based on our hypothesis that the extension lag was due to a restricting adhesion. Because it was now about 8 weeks postsurgery, we felt that maturation of the scar at the repair site provided sufficient tensile strength to allow resistive extension.

> Don't make the reader speculate!

The authors' explanation for why intervention was changed is an important part of case reports. Without an adequate explanation, the reader can only speculate as to why intervention might have been altered.

How Did You *Apply* the Intervention?

In addition to explaining why the intervention was selected and why it changed over time, authors must describe how the intervention was applied—so clearly and completely that another therapist could replicate the intervention with a similar patient. Interventions described in case reports appear primarily in text format, tables or figures, or both. The challenge is to determine which formats will do the best job of operationally defining your interventions.

Steffen[13(p1083)] wrote a clear operational definition of the intervention applied to a patient with mixed progressive supranuclear palsy and corticobasal degeneration. This is only an excerpt, but the authors' use of operational definitions still is clear:

The client trained by walking in each of 4 directions on a Marquette Series 2000 treadmill supported by a Biodex Offset Unweighting System set to unweight 10% of body weight. The sequence of walking direction (forward, backward, left, and right) was randomly determined at each session. To optimize the locomotion training, verbal or tactile feedback was given for proper upright posture while walking. The treadmill had a support bar in front of and to both sides of the client. He was instructed to use the bars to catch his balance, if needed, but to let his arms hang free as often as possible. The treadmill surface was set at a 0% grade, and the speed was increased until the client felt that he was at a safe comfortable pace. The walking time for each direction varied based on client tolerance. On average, the client was walking forward and backward for approximately 6 minutes in each direction at a speed of 2.3 km/h and 1.6 km/h, respectively. Walking sideways was much more difficult for the client. He achieved 6 minutes each way at 1.0 km/h. His heart rate varied from 80 to 120 bpm during sessions. Between walking in each direction, the client took standing rests on the treadmill.

These authors defined the intervention programs more thoroughly later in the manuscript and outlined interventions over a period of $2^1/_2$ years. They also provided data that described the extent of the patient's participation in the intervention.

Some clinical decisions can relate to very specific parts of an intervention, so the intervention description must be just as specific. Olney and colleagues[14(p866)] described use of biofeedback and a gait analysis system with a patient who had a gait disturbance:

> We instructed the patient that a sound would be heard each time she reached the target value within the prescribed phase of the gait cycle and that the feedback coach would give her a score after each six-stride walk. After a few trials, Mrs P was able to obtain the beep with each stride, but she accomplished it by using an exaggerated flexion synergy, elevating her pelvis, and flexing her hip to accomplish the knee flexion. The physical therapist instructed her to allow her pelvis to drop rather than to elevate it and to lift her heel and allow her knee to bend before her forefoot left the ground. She was told that the beep should occur soon after this movement. The target value was decreased from 5 degrees to 3 degrees over the average maximum degrees of flexion to make the task easier. She did not use the abnormal pattern after this instruction.

In their case report of a patient following surgery for a grade III acroioclavicular joint separation, Culp and Romani[15(p864-865)] gave detailed information about the intervention over a 21-week period. Here is an excerpt from weeks 9 through 13:

> In order to strengthen the scapular stabilizing muscles, closed-chain exercises and assisted exercises for the lower trapezius and serratus anterior muscles were initiated. With the patient in the prone manual muscle testing position for the lower trapezius muscle,[26] the physical therapist elevated the patient's arm and assisted him in holding that position for 5 seconds or as long as he could maintain the scapula in the correct position on the thorax. The patient also worked on strengthening at home by placing his arm at about 130 degrees of abduction with the shoulder externally rotated and contracting the lower trapezius muscle to facilitate scapula depression and prevent anterior tilting. Additional strengthening techniques during this period included manual resistance to the scapula to improve the patient's control of adduction and depression. Closed-chain scapular exercises including the push-up "plus" from a wall or floor (Fig. 3), shoulder extension in standing with (minimal) resistance supplied via a Pro Fitter Trainer,[1] (Fig. 4), partial weight bearing through the left upper extremity onto a Swiss ball with the patient bent over at the waist (Fig. 5), and weight bearing through the upper extremity to maintain a Swiss ball on the wall at shoulder height (Fig. 5). [46,47]

To further illustrate their intervention, Culp and Romani[15] provided pictures of the strengthening exercises (the figures mentioned in the text refer to the pictures). They also could have provided videoclips of the physical therapist instructing the patient in how to perform the exercises, which would be helpful to clinicians who want to see exactly how something was done so that they can replicate it.

Patient Participation

Patient participation is an important issue to address in all case reports that describe the implementation of interventions. ("Participation" is preferred to "adherence" or "compliance" because it better reflects the partnership that should exist between patient and therapist.)

TABLE 14. Individual Compliance With Treatment Protocol Over the 5-Week Training Program

Patient No.	No. of Physical Therapy Sessions	Mean Duration of Treatment (min)	Total Treatment Time (h)	% SGT[a]
101	43	56.4	40.42	25.0
106	48	50.9	40.72	27.2
108	50	47.6	39.67	35.5
113	50	52.4	43.67	40.5
201	41	55.8	38.13	28.0
205	39	49.3	32.05	15.7
208	50	55.3	46.10	25.1
211	47	44.5	34.86	40.4
212	50	57.5	47.92	32.5
$\overline{X}$	46.8	52.2	40.39	30.0
SD	4.5	4.5	5.1	8.1
Range	39–50	44.5–57.5	32.1–47.9	15.7–40.5
Maximum value possible	50	60	50	100
% of maximum value	93.6	87	80	30

[a]Percentage of treatment time devoted to special gait training activities.

Reprinted from Malouin F, Potvin M, Prévost J, et al. Use of an intensive task-oriented gait training program in a series of patients with acute cerebrovascular accidents. Phys Ther. 1992;72:781-793; Table 3.

Malouin et al[16] devoted an entire section in their report to this issue, summarizing in a table the data that described the frequency and duration of intervention (Table 14). Sometimes a brief description of a patient's report is all that is needed. The patient could be asked, for example, to keep a daily log of the number of times an exercise program was done. The log should then be used to describe how frequently a patient reported exercising.

In their case report, Sun et al[17] described the use of a daily log to track the home activities included in a constraint-induced movement therapy intervention with their patient who had upper extremity hemiparesis following stroke:

> The treatment diary is a detailed daily log to track use of the affected arm when away from the hospital. The diary was kept to document device use time, as well as activities performed during restraint hours. The patient used this diary for daily documentation and included as much detail and description as possible. For example, the patient might have reported that for the previous day's dinner he ate 80% of a meatball with a built-up spoon. The patient also might report how much time it took to perform an activity, such as 8 minutes to open the door using only the affected upper extremity. The diary assists with ongoing evaluation of program adherence.

An issue related to patient participation is whether the planned intervention was actually carried out. A patient may carry out a home exercise program but might be doing the exercises incorrectly. Descriptions that address both the extent of participation and the correctness of application strengthen a case report.

The case report by Johnson[18 (p671)] illustrates how a patient's home exercise program can be operationally defined. The patient had osteochondritis dissecans (OCD) of the knee:

Ask yourself, "Was the planned intervention actually carried out?"

> A home exercise program was initiated to address the decreased muscle performance of the right lower extremity. The exercises included modified heel slides and modified straight-leg-raising exercises. Modified heel slides (30°–90°) were used to promote pain relief and tissue healing through increased synovial fluid diffusion. Range of motion limits at the knee were used to avoid stress to the lesion site. Modified straight-leg-raising exercises were performed with the knee held in approximately 30 degrees of flexion. Single-plane hip flexion (in a supine position), extension (in a prone position), abduction (in a left side-lying position), and adduction (in a right side-lying position) were performed within full available hip ROM for 2 sets of 10 repetitions each. These exercises were chosen to strengthen the 2-joint muscles that cross the hip and knee joints, to allow for improved load attenuation by these muscles (ie, rectus femoris, hamstring group, gracilis, and tensor fasciae latae/iliotibial band).[28] The decision to perform these exercises with the knee fixed in 30 degrees of flexion was an effort to protect the OCD lesion from further loading while initiating strengthening exercises on day 1 of her intervention.

Home exercise programs commonly are described in case reports. The home exercise program described above illustrates one way of operationalizing a home program. Johnson[18] defined the type of exercises that were done, the rationale for each, the patient's positioning, and the number of repetitions for each exercise. Authors can enhance an operational definition of a home program by describing the patient position during exercise and the amount and type of resistance used. Editors, reviewers, and instructors ask for those details. Again, videoclips can help.

Dunbar[19] operationally defined a home program that was carried out by the mother of a child with sensory processing problems. Dunbar discussed the type of involvement that the mother was able to provide, taking her other obligations into consideration. The mother agreed to take Sara to the park at least once daily for 1 hour, and she agreed to integrate other sensory activities into her daily caregiving routine. Several types of vestibular and proprioceptive activities that Sara seemed to need were available at the park, including monkey-bar climbing, slide play, and games incorporating running and jumping. Dunbar then went on to describe other types of activities that were incorporated into daily activities.

Using Tables and Figures to Summarize

The use of a table to summarize interventions is advantageous for 2 reasons. First, the reader can see the "big picture" when interventions are summarized in a table. Descriptions of interventions in a text format sometimes are difficult to follow, especially when the descriptions are lengthy. Second, the use of a table allows the reader to easily follow the chronology of

TABLE 15. Outline of Home Exercise Program Throughout Physical Therapy Intervention, With Data Compiled From Patient's Daily Exercise Log

	Sets × Repetitions		
	Post-op Weeks 7–8	Post-op Weeks 9–13	Post-op Weeks 14–17
AROM			
Scaption–mirror feedback	1 × 20	1 × 20	
Scapular clock (12, 3, 6, 9)	1 × 10 each direction	1 × 10 each direction	
PROM			
Supine flexion	1 × 20	1 × 20	
ER (shoulder 0° ABD)	1 × 20	1 × 20	
ER (Shoulder 30° ABD)	1 × 20	1 × 20 (60° shoulder ABD)	1 × 20 (90° shoulder ABD)
Side-lying IR		3 × 20 s	3 × 20 s
Codmans	1.4 kg × 2 min		
Prone flexion			20 × 3 s
Shoulder isometrics			
ER	2 × 10 × 5 s	2 × 10 × 5 s	End range 2 × 10 × 5 s
IR	2 × 10 × 5 s	2 × 10 × 5 s	
Flexion	2 × 10 × 5 s	2 × 10 × 5 s	
Extension	2 × 10 × 5 s	2 × 10 × 5 s	
ABD	2 × 10 × 5 s	2 × 10 × 5 s	
Adduction	2 × 10 × 5 s	2 × 10 × 5 s	
Scapular depression	2 × 10 × 5 s	2 × 10 × 5 s	
Scapular retraction	2 × 10 × 5 s	2 × 10 × 5 s	
AROM, Thera-Band			
Wrist flexion	Green 2 × 20	Green 2 × 20	Blue 3 × 15
Wrist extension	Green 2 × 20	Green 2 × 20	Blue 3 × 15
Radial deviation	Green 2 × 20	Green 2 × 20	Blue 3 × 15
Pronation	Green 2 × 20	Green 2 × 20	Blue 3 × 15
Supination	Green 2 × 20	Green 2 × 20	Blue 3 × 15
Elbow flexion	3 × 12 × 3.6 kg	3 × 15 × 4.5 kg	
Elbow extension	3 × 12 × 3.6 kg	3 × 15 × 4.5 kg	
Cane pronation/supination	20	20	
Push-up plus	2 × 10 (hands table height)	2 × 10 (hands to floor)	2 × 12 (feet elevated 15.2 cm)
Swiss ball, UE support			
Bent at waist	2 × 1 min	2 × 1 min	2 × 1 min
Ball at shoulder height			2 × 1 min
AROM patterns			
Saw		1 × 20	1 × 20
Behind back		1 × 20	1 × 20
Behind head		1 × 20	1 × 20
Across shoulder		1 × 20	1 × 20
Overhead		1 × 20	1 × 20
Sport cord decline		Black 3 × 12	
Shrugs			3 × 15 × 4.54 kg
Cable column			
Elbow flexion			3 × 10 × 27.2 kg
Elbow extension			3 × 10 × 31.8 kg
Decline row			3 × 12 × 27.2 kg
Prone shoulder extension/ER			2 × 10 × 2 s
Horizontal ABD			2 × 10 × 2 s
Ball catch release (90° shoulder flexion)			2 × 30 s × 0.9 kg

Post-op=postoperative, AROM=active range of motion, PROM=passive range of motion, ER=external rotation, IR=internal rotation, UE=upper extremity, ABD=abduction

Reprinted from Culp LB, Romani WA. Physical therapist examination, evaluation, and intervention following the surgical reconstruction of a grade III acromioclavicular joint separation. Phys Ther. 2006;86:857-869; Table 2.

intervention. For some examples of how tables and figures have been used in published case reports, see the following pages.

Table 15 contains a home program summary from Culp and Romani's[15] case report on a patient following surgery for a grade III acromioclavicular joint separation. At a glance, the reader can determine how many types of interventions were used, what the interventions were, the number of repetitions the patient did of each exercise, and the amount of resistance. One

TABLE 16. Clinical Reasoning for Rehabilitation Following Shoulder Hemiarthroplasty With Biologic Resurfacing

Period	Short-Term Goals	Clinical Challenge/Decision	Modifications to Rehabilitation Program
Initial evaluation to 6 wk postsurgery	Increase passive ROM	Subscapularis precautions apply, based on surgical procedure	No ER stretching
	Initiate rotator cuff and scapular exercise		No IR resistive exercise
		Meniscal allograft requires healing/incorporation	Use of physiological mobilization in all planes within appropriate ROM restriction (limited ER)
			Limited or no use of accessory glides or shear forces secondary to meniscal allograft incorporation onto glenoid fossa. Minimize translational shear in all rehabilitation activities
		Severe weakness and loss of scapular control	Initiation of early posterior rotator cuff and scapular strengthening/activation exercises. IR exercise and perturbation exercises that engage the subscapularis cannot be used during this period
		Upper trapezius compensation during ADL and any elevation attempts	Use of shortened lever arms during resistive exercise
			Focus on ER movement pattern
			Use of gravity eliminated 90° elevated balance point position to minimize compensation in supine
6 to 14 wk postsurgery	Increase PROM/AROM all planes	Subscapularis precautions stopped at 6 wk postsurgery	Initiate ER stretching in multiple positions of shoulder abduction
	Improve rotator cuff and scapular strength/ stabilization		Advance rotator cuff strengthening program to include IR exercises
	Improve functional elevation for performance of against-gravity tasks		Utilize elevation assistance exercise to minimize compensation from the upper trapezius. Supporting arm on wall against exercise ball or use of supportive sling to slightly unweight extremity are applied during this time frame
	Gain independence with home exercise program	Isometric testing shows significant deficits in IR and ER strength	Continued emphasis on IR and ER strengthening using exercises that can be replicated at home with elastic exercise and light weights. Use of oscillation exercise to increase the number of repetitions of activation also applied
14 wk postsurgery	Prepare for discharge from formal physical therapy	Lack of compliance with traditional home exercise program	Provide all materials and written instruction for rotator cuff and scapular exercise program
			Provide patient with specific recommendations on limiting overhead work and overhead recreational activities for joint preservation

Abbreviations: ADL, activities of daily living; AROM, active range of motion; ER, external rotation; IR, internal rotation; PROM, passive range of motion; ROM, range of motion

Reproduced from Ellenbecker TS, Bailie DS, Lamprecht D. Humeral resurfacing hemiarthroplasty with meniscal allograft in a young patient with glenohumeral osteoarthritis. J Orthop Sports Phys Ther. 2008;38:277-286, Table 3, with permission of the Orthopaedic and Sports Physical Therapy Sections of the American Physical Therapy Association.

TABLE 17. Teleconferencing Technology

Facility	Tele clinic	Conferencing equipment	Max frame rate	Display	Connection types used, rates		
					ISDN	IP	GOES 2 Satellite
SKRI	MTI, PRI	Polycom^{TM} ViewStation MP	30 fps	Single 32" Sony monitor	128–384 kbps	128–768 kbps	PACRIM
NRH	PRI	Polycom^{TM} ViewStation FX	30 fps	Dual 32" Sony monitors	128–384 kbps	128–384 kbps	PACRIM
ELEAH	MTI	Polycom^{TM} ViewStation MP	30 fps	Dual 32" Panasonic monitors	Not supported	128–512 kbps over IP network*	
LBJ	PRI	Polycom^{TM} ViewStation MP	30 fps	Single 32" Sony monitor	128–384 kbps	Not supported	PACRIM

*Optimal connection is at 256 kbps with an ancillary audio (telephone) connection.
Key: SKRI, Sister Kenny Rehabilitation Institute, Minneapolis, MN; NRH, National Rehabilitation Hospital, Washington, DC; ELEAH, ELEAH Medical Center, Elbow Lake, MN; LBJ, Lyndon Baines Johnson Tropical Medical Center, Pago Pago, American Samoa; ISDN, Integrated Digital Services Network; IP, Internet protocol; GOES, Geostationary Orbiting Environmental Satellite.

Reprinted from NeuroRehabilitation; Vol. 18, Savard L, Borstad A, Tkachuck J, et al. Telerehabilitation consultations for clients with neurologic diagnoses: cases from rural Minnesota and American Samoa. Pages 93-102, copyright 2003, with permission from IOS Press.

problem with describing interventions in tabular format is that the descriptions are too brief. Culp and Romani solved that problem by supplementing the table with information in the text.

Ellenbecker and colleagues[20] created a different type of table to report an intervention approach used for a young patient with glenohumeral osteoarthritis who had humeral resurfacing hemiarthroplasty with meniscal allograft (Table 16). The table lists the time post surgery and the short term goals, the "clinical challenge/decision," and modifications of the intervention during each time period. Again, the authors supplemented the information in the table with descriptions in the text.

In a case report written by Savard et al,[21] a table was created to summarize the types of teleconferencing technology used by the different facilities participating in their telerehabilitation consultations for patients with neurologic conditions (Table 17). This is an example of details of an "intervention" in a case report that's not about a patient; the authors further described the intervention in the narrative.

Weeks Postinjury	Treatment	PROM (°)		
		Flexion	Abduction[a]	Lateral Rotation[b]
0	Fracture/dislocation			
6	Moist heat, ultrasound, pendulum, low-grade manual therapy, ice post-exercise (visits three times per week)	80	60	5
6+day	Increase to high-grade manual therapy, continuous passive motion, home program (three times per day): pendulum, wand, ice	80	60	5
8	Allow gentle activities of daily living	100	75	15
10	Reduce visits to twice per week, discontinue ultrasound, add elevation splint 1 hour four times per day	105	85	20
12	Discontinue all treatment in clinic, continue to monitor outcome of home program, add strengthening, increase splint time to 2 hours four times per day	130	105	40
13	No change	140	120	50
14	No change	155	145	65
15	No change	165	160	65
16	No change	165	165	70
25	Patient discharged	175	170	80

[a]Abduction measured with the arm 40° to the coronal plane.
[b]Lateral rotation measured with the arm by the side.

Reprinted from McClure P, Flowers K. Treatment of limited shoulder motion: a case study based on biomechanical considerations. Phys Ther. 1992;72:929-936.

McClure and Flowers[22] used a table to summarize the chronological progression of the intervention and the changes in status in a patient with limited glenohumeral range of motion following a fracture and dislocation of the humeral head (Table 18).

Lowry et al[23] used a table to operationally define the exercises that they used with their patients with patellofemoral pain syndrome (Table 19).

TABLE 19. Exercise Descriptions

Non-Weight-Bearing Exercises	Description
1. Abdominal isometric bracing in hook lying	1. Patient in hook lying and asked to draw lower abdomen inward toward the spine to hold an isometric contraction for 10 s per repetition
a. Abdominal bracing with heel slide	a. Abdominal bracing as above, while sliding heel away from gluteals
b. Abdominal bracing with bent knee lifts	b. Abdominal bracing as above, while performing hip and knee flexion
c. Abdominal bracing with straight-leg raise	c. Abdominal bracing as above, while performing a straight-leg raise
2. Bridging	2. Patient in hook lying and asked to perform abdominal bracing, while lifting gluteals from the table
3. Side-lying clamshells	3. Patient in side lying, with hip and knees flexed at 45°. Patient lifts upper most knee toward the ceiling, while keeping the feet together
4. Quadruped upper extremity shoulder flexion and lower extremity hip extension	4. Patient in quadruped and asked to perform abdominal bracing, while simultaneously lifting opposite upper and lower extremity
5 Quadruped lower extremity abduction and extension	5. Patient in quadruped and asked to perform abdominal bracing, while simultaneously abducting and extending hip with knee in flexion

Weight-Bearing Exercises	Description
1. Double-leg press	1. Patient on Total Gym machine and asked to simultaneously flex hip and knee to squat bilaterally
2. Single-leg press	2 Patient on Total Gym machine and asked to simultaneously flex hip and knee to squats unilaterally
3. Eccentric step-downs from step	3. Patient standing on small 10-cm step, facing forward, and asked to eccentrically lower opposite heel from the step, progressed by raising height of step
4. Eccentric side step-downs from step	4. Patient standing on small 10-cm step, facing side, and asked to eccentrically lower opposite heel from the step, progressed by raising height of step
5. Hip abduction sidestepping, with resistive band at ankles	5. Patient standing, with resistive band wrapped around ankles, and asked to slightly flex knees and hips, while sidestepping against resistance
6. Squats	6. Patient standing and asked to simultaneously flex knees and hips to perform partial squat, progressed by performing deeper squats
7. Lunge	7. Patient standing with one lower extremity in front of the other and asked to flex hip and knee of forward most lower extremity to perform a lunge
8. Clock balance and reach[†]	8. Patient standing on affected lower extremity with knee slightly flexed. Patient asked to reach with opposite heel directly in front of the affected lower extremity (12:00) and then to reach forward and to the side (1:00) and so forth in a circle.[†]

Stretches	Description
1. Supine piriformis stretch	1. Patient in supine, with affected knee flexed and crossed over the other. Stretch was performed gently pulling affected knee toward opposite shoulder
2. Supine gluteus figure-four stretch	2. Patient in supine, with affected knee flexed and crossed over the other. Stretch was performed gently pushing knee downward
3. Standing hamstrings stretch	3. Patient in standing, with knee extended and hip flexed, with foot resting on step. Stretch was performed by leaning forward to stretch hamstring, while maintaining anterior pelvic tilt
4. Standing quadriceps stretch	4. Patient in standing, with knee flexed and hip in neutral. Stretch ws performed by pulling heel toward gluteal
5. Standing iliotibial band/tensor fascia lata stretch	5. Patient in standing, with affected lower extremity behind other lower extremity, with knee and hip extended. Stretch was performed by leaning away from the affected lower extremity
6. Standing gastrocnemius/soleus stretch	6. Patient in standing, with affected lower extremity behind other lower extremity, with knee and hip extended. Stretch was performed by flexing foremost knee, while keeping rearmost heel on the floor.

* Exercises were commenced after manual therapy treatment and prescribed for home once they were performed correctly in the clinic. Exercises were individualized for each patient and performed 1-2 times per day.

† Adapted from Loudon et al.[44]

Reproduced from Lowry CD, Cleland JA, Dyke K. Management of patients with patellofemoral pain syndrome using a multimodal approach: a case series. J Orthop Sports Phys Ther. 2008;38:691-702, Table 3, with permission of the Orthopaedic and Sports Physical Therapy Sections of the American Physical Therapy Association.

FIGURE 28. Single-leg standing activities with perturbations. The patient was instructed to hold on to the Thera-Band at the level of the umbilicus, and oscillating perturbations were applied by the therapist pulling on the Thera-Band. Perturbations can be applied in multiple directions and at various speeds and intensities.

Reprinted from Helgeson K, Smith AR Jr. Process for applying the *International Classification of Functioning, Disability and Health* model to a patient with patellar dislocation. *Phys Ther.* 2008;88:956-964; Figure 7.

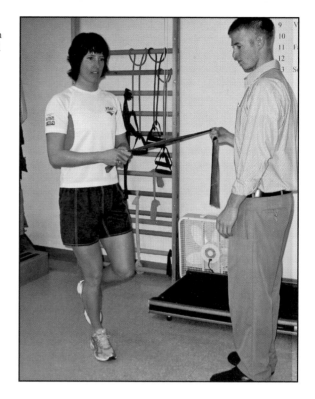

Helgeson and Smith[27] included a photograph in their case report to clarify the operational definitions of an exercise that was used for a patient with a diagnosis of patellar dislocation (Figure 28).

Using Appendixes to Provide Specific Information

Appendixes also can be used to provide information about interventions. Cook et al[28] used an appendix to describe one of the components of dressing training for elderly patients with cognitive and perceptual impairments (Figure 29).

Audiotape Script for Dressing Training

Time	Cue	Instruction
	1	"Ethel, listen to the tape. It is time to dress."
	2	"Look at your bed. Do not touch your clothes until told to do so by the tape."
12 sec	3	"Take off your nightgown."
5 sec	4	"Put your nightgown on your bed BEHIND your pile of clothes."
1 min 30 sec	5	"Pick up your bra. Put it on."
1 min 50 sec	6	"Put on your blouse [slight pause] and button it."
45 sec	7	"Put on your underpants."
1 min 40 sec	8	"Put on your pants."
50 sec	9	"Take ONE sock and put it on."
50 sec	10	"Take the other sock and put it on."
60 sec	11	"Take ONE shoe. Put it on and tie it."
60 sec	12	"Take the other shoe. Put it on and tie it."
	13	"STOP. Make sure you have put on all of your clothes. Check your bra. Check your blouse. Check your pants. Check your left sock. Check your right sock. Check your left shoe. Check your right shoe."
	14	"You are finished dressing. STOP."

FIGURE 29. An appendix used to provide information about a specific component of an intervention.

Used with permission of *Am J Occup Ther*. 45:652-654; 1991 Cook EA, Luschen L, Sikes S. Dressing training for an elderly woman with cognitive and perceptual impairments; permission conveyed through Copyright Clearance Center Inc.

NEXT

What Happened?

"Outcomes" are more than changes in the patient's impairments, such as range of motion. Case reports should include changes in the patient's ability to do those things that are important to that patient—getting dishes out of a cabinet, walking to the bathroom. There are many ways to depict outcomes. Be creative!

References

1 Guide to Physical Therapist Practice. 2nd ed. *Phys Ther.* 2001;81:9-744. Revised 2003.

2 Occupational therapy practice framework: domain and process, ed 2. *Am J Occup Ther.* 2008; 62:625–683.

3 Dalton GW, Keating JL. Number needed to treat: a statistic relevant for physical therapists. *Phys Ther.* 2000;80:1214-1219.

4 Cohen J. *Statistical Power Analysis for the Behavioral Sciences.* 2nd ed. Hillsdale, NJ: Lawrence Erlbaum Associates; 1988.

5 Newman D, Allison SC. Risk and physical therapy? *J Orthop Sports Phys Ther.* 2007;37:287-289.

6 Straus SE, Richardson WS, Glasziou P, Haynes RB. *Evidence-based Medicine: How to Practice and Teach EBM.* 3rd ed. New York, NY: Churchill Livingstone; 2005.

7 Portney LG, Watkins MP. *Foundations of Clinical Research: Applications to Practice.* 3rd ed. Upper Saddle River, NJ: Prentice Hall; 2009.

8 Vaughn DW. Isolated knee pain: a case report highlighting regional interdependence. *J Orthop Sports Phys Ther.* 2008;38:616-623.

9 Deutsch JE, Borbely M, Filler J, et al. Use of a low-cost, commercially available gaming console (Wii) for rehabilitation of an adolescent with cerebral palsy. *Phys Ther.* 2008;88:1196-1207.

10 Schenkman, Hall D, Kumar R, Kohrt KM. Endurance exercise training to improve economy of movement of people with Parkinson disease: three case reports. *Phys Ther.* 2008;88:63-76.

11 Carlson M, Hadlock T. Physical therapist management following rotator cuff repair for a patient with postpolio syndrome. *Phys Ther.* 2007;87:179-192.

12 Flowers KR, McClure PW, McFadden C. Management of a patient with lacerations of the tendons of the extensor digitorum and extensor indicis muscles to the index finger. *Phys Ther.* 1996;76: 61-67.

13 Steffen TM, Boeve BF, Mollinger-Riemann LA, Petersen CM. Long-term locomotor training for gait and balance in a patient with mixed progressive supranuclear palsy and corticobasal degeneration. *Phys Ther.* 2007;87:1078-1087.

14 Olney SJ, Colbourne GR, Martin CS. Joint angle biofeedback and biomechanical gait analysis in stroke patients: a case report. *Phys Ther.* 1989;69:863-870.

15 Culp LB, Romani WA. Physical therapist examination, evaluation, and intervention following the surgical reconstruction of a grade III acromioclavicular joint separation. *Phys Ther.* 2006;86:857-869.

16 Malouin F, Potvin M, Prévost J, et al. Use of an intensive task-oriented gait training program in a series of patients with acute cerebrovascular accidents. *Phys Ther.* 1992;72:781-793.

17 Sun SF, Hsu CW, Hwang CW, et al. Application of combined botulinum toxin type A and modified constraint-induced movement therapy for an individual with chronic upper-extremity spasticity after stroke. *Phys Ther.* 2006;86:1387-1397.

18 Johnson MP. Physical therapist management of an adult with osteochondritis dissecans of the knee. *Phys Ther.* 2005;85:665-675.

19 Dunbar SB. A child's occupational performance: considerations of sensory processing and family context. *Am J Occup Ther.* 1999;53:231-235.

20 Ellenbecker TS, Bailie DS, Lamprecht D. Humeral resurfacing hemiarthroplasty with meniscal allograft in a young patient with glenohumeral osteoarthritis. *J Orthop Sports Phys Ther.* 2008;38:277-286.

21 Savard L, Borstad A, Tkachuck J, et al. Telerehabilitation consultations for clients with neurologic diagnoses: cases from rural Minnesota and American Samoa. *NeuroRehabilitation.* 2003;18:93-102.

22 McClure P, Flowers K. Treatment of limited shoulder motion: a case study based on biomechanical considerations. *Phys Ther.* 1992;72:929-936.

23 Lowry CD, Cleland JA, Dyke K. Management of patients with patellofemoral pain syndrome using a multimodal approach: a case series. *J Orthop Sports Phys Ther.* 2008;38:691-702.

24 Twist DJ. Acrocyanosis in a spinal cord injured patient—effects of computer-controlled neuromuscular electrical stimulation: a case report. *Phys Ther.* 1990;70:45-49.

25 Johnson J, Silverberg R. Serial casting of the lower extremity to correct contractures during the acute phase of burn care. *Phys Ther.* 1995;75:262-266.

26 Dunning K, Berberich A, Albers B, et al. A four-week, task-specific neuroprosthesis program for a person with no active wrist or finger movement because of chronic stroke. *Phys Ther.* 2008;88:397-405.

27 Helgeson K, Smith AR Jr. Process for applying the International Classification of Functioning, Disability and Health model to a patient with patellar dislocation. *Phys Ther.* 2008;88:956-964.

28 Cook EA, Luschen L, Sikes S. Dressing training for an elderly woman with cognitive and perceptual impairments. *Am J Occup Ther.* 1991;45:652-654.

CHAPTER 9

Describing the Outcomes

What is an outcome? It can be how a group of people function in a given environment or it can be the status of patients after an intervention.

For the purpose of a case report, "outcome" is defined as the status of the patient, other entity, or situation following intervention. When the case report describes "nonpatients" (eg, students), the outcome usually relates to how those nonpatients function in the environment described in the report. When the case report describes patients, the outcome usually relates to the patient's ability to complete tasks and engage in life situations (activities and participation). Outcomes also can relate to risk reduction/prevention; health, wellness, and fitness; societal resources; and patient/client satisfaction.[1] Remember: case reports can only describe outcomes; they can't prove that interventions cause outcomes.

Some case reports describe changes in impairments, such as range of motion or pain, as an outcome—but that's not enough. At a minimum, case reports should describe changes that occur in activities and participation. After all, improvement in impairments may not always relate to the aim of intervention, which is to improve a patient's ability to function in real life.

Outcomes can be measured using one or more of the tests and measures designed to assess the patient's ability to function. A review of **Chapter 4 and 5** on measurement and change could be helpful when deciding on outcome measures and writing about them

Focus on the
patient's report
of changes

Although published tests or measures can provide useful information about a patient's change, it is not necessary to use one if the outcome can be better described through the *patient's report* of changes in activities and participation. Some published tests and measures are not responsive enough to detect changes that are meaningful for individual patients; others might not contain items that measure the patient's desired outcomes. Even when published tests and measures are used, case reports are strengthened if the patient's reports of progress are obtained during the course of intervention as well as at the end of intervention and—if long-term follow-up information is obtained—even from a simple telephone call. Outcomes can be depicted in text, tables, or a variety of figures.

Outcomes in Text

Riddle et al[2(p483)] reported the following outcome after an intervention program for a patient with low back pain. They said in part:

> The patient reported that she had achieved all of her goals except she still had some intermittent mild pain when putting on stockings in the morning and when rolling in bed. She rated the intensity of this pain as 1 on the 0 to 10 verbal pain rating scale. She also said that the pain lasted only a few seconds. She stated the pain occurred approximately once every 4 mornings. She appeared to be ready to complete the episode of physical therapy care.

The outcome described by Riddle et al[2] illustrates the importance of reporting on the patient's ability to perform functional activities. Despite improvement in impairments, the patient still had some pain when putting on her stockings and rolling in bed. Although the patient had not achieved all of her goals, the authors decided to discharge her from physical therapy because they believed she would continue to improve by doing exercises in the morning at home. A follow-up phone call might have confirmed this belief.

In her case report of a child with sensory processing problems, Dunbar[3(pp233-234)] first described improvement in impairment, as measured by a standardized test, and then improvement in activities and participation that were important to the child's family:

> Sara had made tremendous gains evidenced by an increase in scores on the DeGangi-Berk Test of Sensory Integration. Her retest score increased by 8 points (from 7 to 15) for postural control, by 17 points (from 4 to 21) for bilateral motor integration, and by 14 points (from 0 to 14) for reflex integration. Specific improvements in Sara's behavior and occupational performance that had meaning for this particular family were an ability to quietly color and engage in other tabletop play for a 2-hour airplane trip, cessation of head banging, diminishment of tantrums, and sleeping though the night.

Another outcome that Dunbar[3] described was Sara's mother's statement that she had an increased awareness of ways in which she could help her daughter. If studies had identified the MDC and MCID of the DeGangi-Berk Test of Sensory Integration with similar children, and if the author had reported it, that information would have helped readers to understand the meaning of the change in the child's scores on the test.

The case report by Rundell and colleagues[4 (pp87-88)] used the ICF framework to describe the physical therapist management of 2 patients with chronic low back pain (LBP). The authors used a variety of methods to measure outcomes over time in the body structures and functions, activity, and participation components of the ICF. This is how they described outcomes for one of the patients:

> Immediate improvement was demonstrated after the initial manipulation, with 0/10 lumbar and leg pain in standing, no pain with lumbar extension AROM, decreased pain with left side-bending AROM, and no pain with right single-leg stance. At the second visit, her right LBP and leg pain were less intense (ie, 2/10 at worst). Extension created right lumbar pain at end-range, and right L5–S1 accessory motion was still painful and hypomobile. She was able to sit 5 hours at work without LBP, and her RMQ [Roland-Morris Disability Questionnaire] score was 1/24. During the final visit, the patient reported no pain since the day of the last treatment. She was working a full day and returned to jogging without pain. Her final RMQ score was 0/24. Her LoBACS [Lower Back Activity Confidence Scale] scores were 91%, 100%, and 100% for the function, self-regulatory, and exercise subscales, respectively. Her FABQ [Fear-Avoidance Belief Questionnaire] scores were 5/42 for the work subscale and 4/24 for the physical activity subscale. Re-examination demonstrated normal lumbar AROM, normal and pain-free accessory motion testing, and a negative slump test. The patient was discharged from physical therapy with all goals met.

Vaughn and Nitsch[5 (p1586)] reported their patient's outcomes both at the time of termination of physical therapy services and at follow-up 1 year later. The patient was a tennis-playing student whose function was limited by ilial anterior rotation hypermobility:

> Goals the patient met in the set time frames included: decreasing the tissue tenderness and tonicity of the right SIJ region comparable to the left side (1–2 weeks); restoring pelvis, lower-extremity, and trunk joint mobility and tissue flexibility comparable to the left side (6–8 weeks); progressing to sacroiliac stabilization exercises (9–10 weeks); progressing to aerobic conditioning exercises (11–14 weeks); and progressing to agility exercises (15–20 weeks). The patient met her long-term goal of returning to competitive tennis at the collegiate level, but not until the 26th week. The results of the tests and measures from the examination and final assessment are recorded in the Table …. The patient graduated at the end of the spring semester and was reexamined 1 year later. No impairments or functional limitations were found on examination, and the patient reported she could perform all of her normal activities pain-free without the sacroiliac belt or proprioceptive taping.

The table that Vaughn and Nitsch[5] mentioned lists the tests and measures that they used, the impairments identified by each during the examination, and the impairments on final assessment. The patient's report of her return to competitive tennis after the 26th week and her ability to carry out all of her activities without pain after 1 year help complete the picture of her functioning following the episode of physical therapy. Linking measurements of impairments in body structures and functions, activity limitations, and participation restrictions gives readers insights into which impairments might be the most relevant to the patient's functioning. Because

N's performance on the GMFM (Gross Motor Function Measure) did improve (Table 2). The improvement corresponded to the four-week time period of increased PT, especially in the lying/rolling and crawling/kneeling domains. Specific items in which N demonstrated improvement included pivoting in prone (items 16 and 17), crawling/hitching forward (item 44), and pulling to stand at a large bench (item 52).

Savard et al[10(pp99-100)] wrote a case report about the development and implementation of a telerehabilitation program for people with neurologic conditions living in Minnesota and American Samoa. Their outcomes section reported program data rather than individual patient outcomes:

A total of 117 telerehabilitation encounters have been completed with 75 patients in our programs since their inception in October of 2000. Thirty-eight of those visits have been for individuals with neurologic diagnoses. Of that set 25 of the visits were for initial assessments, and 13 were follow-up visits. Table 3 includes a breakdown of the numbers of visits by program, type of diagnosis and visit type. The age range of patients was 9 months to 86 years. Ages of participants, by decade, are listed in Table 4. Diagnoses of participants included cerebral vascular accident, Parkinson's disease, spinal cord injury, cerebral palsy, spinal muscular atrophy, traumatic brain injury, amyotrophic lateral sclerosis, multiple sclerosis, muscular dystrophy and shoulder dystocia.

All consultations led to changes to the rehabilitation plan of care. These changes were the result of specialist recommendations regarding exercise programs, adaptive equipment, manual therapy, functional training, cognitive and swallowing interventions, positioning, wound care and medications. Sometimes, additional medical tests were suggested for diagnostic purposes. All of the patients seen in the MTI [Minnesota Telerehabilitation Initiative] program (n = 26) reported good to excellent satisfaction with the visits. Twenty-three patients had positive clinical outcomes. Patients in the PRI [Pacific Rim Initiative] program (n = 49) were not surveyed regarding satisfaction due to cultural issues creating a Rosenthal effect. Nineteen clinicians participated in the projects. Clinicians rated the clinical effectiveness of every specialty teleconsult as good or excellent.

The average mileage saved for MTI participants was 150 miles, one way. For individuals living in American Samoa, specialty rehabilitation services are not available. Specialty services may only be found off the island and could be accessed only when an individual can fund travel and medical expenses privately.

Other case reports that are not directly related to patients, such as case reports about education programs or administrative situations, could report similar kinds of data, such as number of people served and their characteristics and other outcomes related to the goals of the program.

The above excerpts from case reports give examples of outcomes written in narrative form. Tables and figures are other ways to present outcomes; they often are especially useful to succinctly describe outcomes that might be difficult to write about and understand in narrative form. When using tables and figures, avoid giving the same information again in the narrative.

TABLE 20. Metabolic Data From Patient in the Current Case Report Compared With Data From Selected Literature[a]

Study	Group	HR (bpm)	SSWS (m/s)	$\dot{V}O_2$ (mL/kg/min)
Waters et al[9]	Transtibial amputation	106	1.18	15.5
	Transfemoral amputation	111	0.86	12.9
	Control	104	1.36	13.0
Nowroozi et al[8]	Hip disarticulation	99	0.79	11.1
	Hemipelvectomy	97	0.66	11.4
	Control	74	1.25	9.8
Gailey et al[19]	Transtibial amputation	103	1.16	12.9
	Control	87	1.25	10.9
Patient in current case report	Hip disarticulation	131	0.86	14.49

[a] Control groups within the literature represent individuals without amputations. Heart rate (HR) and oxygen consumption ($\dot{V}O_2$) values are reported during steady-state ambulation at self-selected walking speeds (SSWS).

Adapted from Schnall BL, Baum BS, Andrews AM. Gait characteristics of a soldier with a traumatic hip disarticulation. Phys Ther. *2008;88:1568-1577; Table 3.*

A brief summary is fine, but let the table or figure tell most of the story. Never present outcomes *only* in tables or figures, though! Some narrative is necessary to tie them together.

Outcomes in Tables

Several of the descriptions excerpted in this chapter referred to tables. In a table that is unusual, Schnall et al[11] reported metabolic data of their patient with a traumatic hip disarticulation when he was walking at a self-selected speed. For comparison purposes, the table also includes data from 3 studies of people without impairments and people with transtibial and transfemoral amputations, hip disarticulation, and hemipelvectomy (Table 20).

Tables can be particularly useful for summarizing chronological changes in tests and measures over time. Vaughn and Nitsch[5] used a table to summarize changes in tests and measures of their patient's impairments from the initial examination to the final examination (Table 21).

Head and Patterson[12] created a table that concisely summarized their client's problems, the adaptive equipment intervention selected to address each problem, the outcome, and the cost (Table 22).

TABLE 21. Results From Tests and Measures at Examination and Final Assessment

Tests and Measures	Impairments Identified on Examination	Impairments on Final Assessment
Pain intensity level	8/10 in sitting, standing, or walking; 6/10 in left side lying with pillow between knees	0/10 in all positions and activities
Gait analysis	Right antalgic gait pattern	Normal gait pattern
Posture and alignment	Standing: decreased weight bearing on right lower extremity (hip flexed and lateral rotation) Sitting: decreased weight bearing on right pelvis	Good postural alignment in standing and sitting, equal weight bearing
Active mobility testing	Decreased posterior rotation and translation in right innominate	Right posterior rotation and translation comparable to left side
Passive range of motion and end-feel	Right hip flexion 100° (hard end-feel); medial rotation 0° (pain limited); abduction 20° (elastic end-feel)	Right hip flexion 130° (elastic end-feel); medial rotation 35° (firm end feel); abduction 40° (elastic end-feel)
Length tests	Hamstring muscles 60°; piriformis muscle decreased adduction to midline; iliopsoas muscle -30°; rectus femoris muscle 60°; Ober test painful	Hamstring muscles 90°; piriformis muscle adduction past midline; iliopsoas muscle 0° (neutral); rectus femoris muscle 90°; negative Ober test
Passive mobility testing	Right ilial posterior rotation grade 1 (hard end-feel); ilial anterior rotation grade 5 (loose end-feel), correction of positional fault	Right ilial posterior rotation grade 3 (firm end-feel); ilial anterior rotation grade 3 (firm end-feel), reexamined 1 y later
Palpation	Increased temperature and tenderness of right long dorsal sacral iliac ligament; hypertonicity of right piriformis, erector spinae, and iliopsoas muscles	Normal temperature and tenderness of right long dorsal sacral iliac ligament; normal tonicity of right piriformis, erector spinae, and iliopsoas muscle
Special tests	Positive FABER, Ostgaard, and long-sit tests; apparent leg length discrepancy	Negative FABER, Ostgaard, and long-sit tests; equal leg lengths

Reprinted from Vaughn HT, Nitsch W. Ilial anterior rotation hypermobility in a female collegiate tennis player. Phys Ther. 2008;88:1578-1590; Table

TABLE 22. Summary of Interventions

Problem	Intervention	Outcome	Cost
Unsafe, limited mobility	Powered wheelchair	Trial use—not accepted by client because he did not feel safe	Loaner from stock
	Lightweight manual wheelchair	Independent in indoor mobility	$360
Limited bed mobility	Electric hospital bed	Independent	$650
Inaccessible home entrance	Wheelchair ramp	Able to enter and exit home with assistance	$1200
Unable to open containers	Loop scissors, tab gripper, jar lid opener	Used infrequently	$20
Difficulty with feeding and drinking	Long straw, lightweight cup with handle, nonskid mat	Able to perform activities with greater ease	$40
Unable to wear shoes	Special booties	Increased warmth and protection from trauma	$50
Difficulty holding toothbrush	Tubing to build up handle	Independent	$3
Unable to pick up objects from floor	Dressing stick	Used to pick up some items (e.g., clothing) and to extend reach	$10

Used with permission of Am J Occup Ther. 1997;51:453-457. Head J, Patterson V. Performance context and its role in treatment planning; permission conveyed through Copyright Clearance Center Inc.

Changes in COPM Ratings

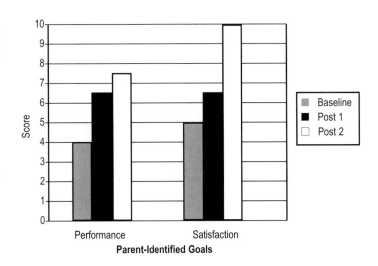

FIGURE 30. Changes in the mean performance and satisfaction ratings of parent-identified goals from preintervention (baseline) to immediate postintervention (Post 1) and 3 months postintervention (Post 2). COPM=Canadian Occupational Performance Measure.

Used with permission of *Am J Occup Ther.* 62(3):282-288;2008 May-June; Figure 1. Martin A, Burtner PA, Poole J, Phillips J. Case report: ICF-level changes in a preschooler after constraint-induced movement therapy.; permission conveyed through Copyright Clearance Center Inc.

AROM Measurements

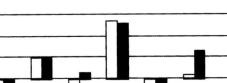

	CMC thumb Abduction	MCP Ext. 2nd	MCP Ext. 5th	Wrist Flexion	Wrist Extension	Elbow Flexion	Elbow Extension	Forearm Supination	Shoulder Flexion
Pretest	−20	−30	−35	50	−50	135	−15	10	0
Posttest	50	−60	−60	50	15	130	−15	65	35

FIGURE 31. Active range-of-motion (AROM) measurements before and after repetitive-task practice/Hand Mentor intervention. The patient improved in carpal-metacarpal (CMC) thumb abduction, wrist extension, forearm supination, and shoulder flexion. MCP=metacarpal-phalangeal.

Used with permission of *Am J Occup Ther.* 62(1):28-35;2008 Jan-Feb; Figure 2. Rosenstein L, Ridget AL, Thota A, Samame B, Alberts JL. Effects of combined robotic therapy and repetitive-task practice on upper-extremity function in a patient with chronic stroke; permission conveyed through Copyright Clearance Center Inc.

Outcomes in Histograms

Martin and colleagues[13] used a histogram to show changes in Canadian Occupational Performance Measure ratings by the parent of a child with cerebral palsy who received constraint-induced movement therapy (Figure 30).

Rosenstein and colleagues[14] used a histogram to illustrate changes in the upper-extremity active range of motion of a patient with chronic stroke before and after a combination of robotic therapy using Hand Mentor and repetitive task practice (Figure 31).

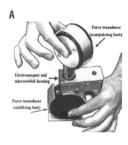

A

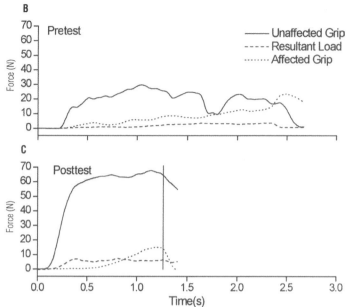

B

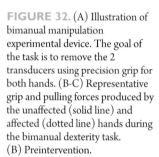

FIGURE 32. (A) Illustration of bimanual manipulation experimental device. The goal of the task is to remove the 2 transducers using precision grip for both hands. (B-C) Representative grip and pulling forces produced by the unaffected (solid line) and affected (dotted line) hands during the bimanual dexterity task. (B) Preintervention. (C) Postintervention. The patient was unable to perform the task before the intervention. In the posttest, however, she was able to produce sufficient grip and pulling forces with appropriate timing to separate the 2 objects. Object separation time is represented by the solid vertical line.

Outcomes in Line Graphs

In addition to using a histogram, Rosenstein et al[14] used a line graph. Figure 32 shows a picture of the device used to measure maximum grip and force loads for both hands when a patient attempted to separate 2 transducers. The figure also shows pretest and posttest forces, which indicated that the patient was unable to separate the transducers initially but at posttest was able to exert grip and pulling forces with appropriate timing to separate the transducers.

In their case report of constraint-induced therapy for a child with cerebral palsy, Martin et al[13] used a line graph to summarize the changes that took place in the child's grip strength before intervention, immediately after intervention, and 3 months after intervention (Figure 33).

Morrison[15] wrote a case report about a patient with quadriplegia who was treated with electromyographic biofeedback. The goal of biofeedback training was to improve his accessory breathing muscle activity and therefore his vital capacity. Figure 34 shows the amount of time that the patient was taken off the ventilator during each intervention session.

Chapter 9: Describing the Outcomes

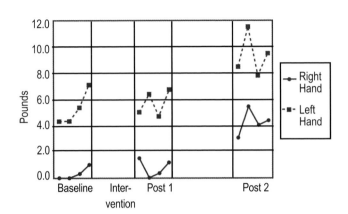

Changes in Grip Strength

FIGURE 33. Changes in mean grip strength for the participant's left (less involved) hand and the right (hemiplegic) hand from preintervention (baseline) to immediate postintervention (Post 1) and 3 months postintervention (Post 2) phases. Note that the measures were taken on 4 different days in each phase. On each day, 3 grip measures were taken and the mean recorded as the data point on this figure.

Used with permission of *Am J Occup Ther.* 62(3):282-288;2008 May-June; Figure 4. Martin A, Burtner PA, Poole J, Phillips J. Case report: ICF-level changes in a preschooler after constraint-induced movement therapy; permission conveyed through Copyright Clearance Center Inc.

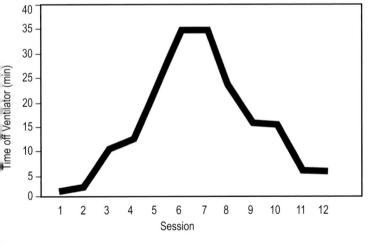

FIGURE 34. Amount of time off mechanical ventilator achieved by patient with high-level quadriplegia during (sessions 1-6) and after (sessions 7-12) electromyographic feedback training.

Reprinted from Morrison SA. Biofeedback to facilitate unassisted ventilation in individuals with high-level quadriplegia: a case report. *Phys Ther.* 1988;68:1378-1380; Figure 3.

FIGURE 35. Involved foot. Hatch marks on a darker background indicate medial column bones with a bone mineral density response lower than that of lateral column bones (hatch marks on a lighter background). Numbers inside bones represent the percentage of change on the involved side from before reloading to after reloading.

Reprinted from Hastings MK, Gelber J, Commean PK, et al. Bone mineral density of the tarsals and metatarsals with reloading. *Phys Ther.* 2008;88:766-779; Figure 2.

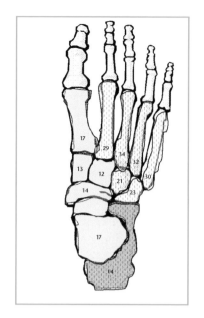

FIGURE 36. Vertical ground reaction force of the prosthetic and intact limbs compared with controls (±2 SD). The gait cycles are normalized to consecutive footstrikes of each limb.

Reprinted from Schnall BL, Baum BS, Andrews AM. Gait characteristics of a soldier with a traumatic hip disarticulation. *Phys Ther.* 2008;88:1568-1577; Figure 4.

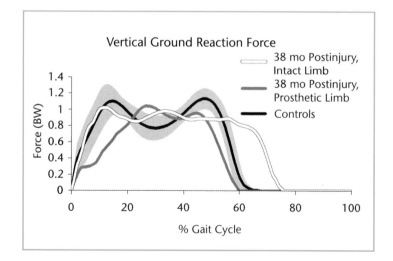

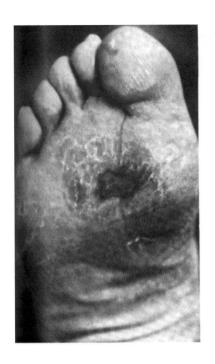

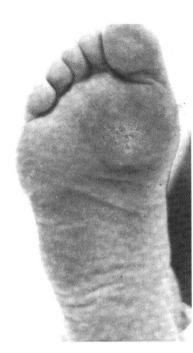

FIGURE 37. (left) Plantar ulcer after treatment with total contact casting for 85 days.

Reprinted from Mueller MJ, Diamond JE. Biomechanical treatment approach to diabetic plantar ulcers: a case report. *Phys Ther.* 1988;68:1917-1920.

FIGURE 38. Plantar surface of patient's foot at 6-month follow-up visit.

Outcomes in Scans and Photographs

Hastings et al[16] wrote a case report to describe changes in the tarsal and metatarsal bone mineral density following a 26-week progressive reloading program for a woman who had been previously been non–weight bearing for 6 weeks. They used quantitative computed tomography to measure bone mineral density (Figure 35).

Schnall et al[11] used gait analysis data to show the vertical ground-reaction forces during ambulation of their patient with a traumatic hip disarticulation compared with control subjects (Figure 36).

Mueller and Diamond[17] used photos of a patient's foot to illustrate the changes that took place in a plantar ulcer that was treated using a total contact cast (Figures 37, 38).

FIGURE 39. Pretreatment radiographic films of right femur of patient with myositis ossificans: (A) anterior-posterior view; (B) lateral view.

Reprinted from Weider DL. Treatment of traumatic myositis ossificans with acetic acid iontophoresis. *Phys Ther.* 1992;72:133-137.

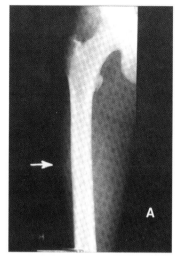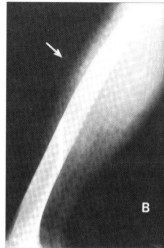

FIGURE 40. Posttreatment radiographic films of right femur of patient with myositis ossificans: (A) anterior-posterior view; (B) lateral view.

Weider DL. Treatment of traumatic myositis ossificans with acetic acid iontophoresis. *Phys Ther.* 1992;72:133-137.

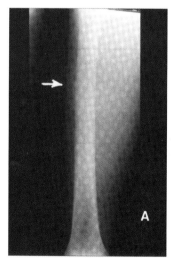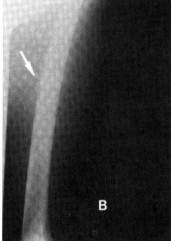

Outcomes in Radiographs

In Wieder's description of the intervention of a patient with a diagnosis of traumatic myositis ossificans,[18] radiographs were used to illustrate the changes that took place in the pathology following a course of intervention (Figures 39, 40).

NEXT

What Does Your Case Report Mean?

Changes in impairments can be important to report, but impairment measurements must be linked to changes in patients' activities and participation. Changes in radiographs, vital capacity, range of motion, developmental test results for children, or foot pressure are not enough. Changes in ability to lift boxes, shop for groceries, take care of children, work at a computer, play sports, or do other activities that are important to patients also must be reported. Once you've done that, it's time to offer possible explanations for what happened in the case.

References

1 Guide to Physical Therapist Practice. 2nd ed. *Phys Ther.* 2001;81:9-744. Revised June 2003.

2 Riddle DL, Rothstein JM, Echternach JL. Application of the HOAC II: an episode of care for a patient with low back pain. *Phys Ther.* 2003;83:471-485.

3 Dunbar SB. A child's occupational performance: considerations of sensory processing and family context. *Am J Occup Ther.* 1999;53:231-235.

4 Rundell SD, Davenport TE, Wagner T. Physical therapist management of acute and chronic low back pain using the World Health Organization's *International Classification of Functioning, Disability and Health. Phys Ther.* 2009;89:82-90.

5 Vaughn HT, Nitsch W. Ilial anterior rotation hypermobility in a female collegiate tennis player. *Phys Ther.* 2008;88:1578-1590

6 Yates C, Bandy WD, Blasier RD. Traumatic dislocation of the hip in a high school football player. *Phys Ther.* 2008;88:780-788.

7 Bellamy SG, Gibbs K, Lazaro R. Physical therapy intervention for an adolescent with a knee flexion contracture and diagnosis of multiple pterygium syndrome. *Pediatr Phys Ther.* 2007;19:140-147.

8 Schenkman M, Hall D, Kumar R, Kohrt WM. Endurance exercise training to improve economy of movement of people with Parkinson disease: three case reports. *Phys Ther.* 2008;88:63-76.

9 Schreiber J. Increased intensity of physical therapy for a child with gross motor developmental delay: a case report. *Phys Occup Ther Pediatr.* 2004;24(4):63-78.

10 Savard L, Borstad A, Tkachuck J, et al. Telerehabilitation consultations for clients with neurologic diagnoses: cases from rural Minnesota and American Samoa. *NeuroRehabilitation.* 2003;18:93-102.

11 Schnall BL, Baum BS, Andrews AM. Gait characteristics of a soldier with a traumatic hip disarticulation. *Phys Ther.* 2008;88:1568-1577.

12 Head J, Patterson V. Performance context and its role in treatment planning. *Am J Occup Ther.* 1997;51:453-457.

13 Martin A, Burtner PA, Poole J, Phillips J. Case report: ICF-level changes in a preschooler after constraint-induced movement therapy. *Am J Occup Ther.* 2008;62:282-288.

14 Rosenstein L, Ridgel AL, Thota A, et al. Effects of combined robotic therapy and repetitive-task practice on upper extremity function in a patient with chronic stroke. *Am J Occup Ther.* 2008;62:28-35.

15 Morrison SA. Biofeedback to facilitate unassisted ventilation in individuals with high-level quadriplegia: a case report. *Phys Ther.* 1988;68:1378-1380.

16 Hastings MK, Gelber J, Commean PK, et al. Bone mineral density of the tarsals and metatarsals with reloading. *Phys Ther.* 2008;88:766-779.

17 Mueller MJ, Diamond JE. Biomechanical treatment approach to diabetic plantar ulcers: a case report. *Phys Ther.* 1988;68:1917-1920.

18 Weider DL. Treatment of traumatic myositis ossificans with acetic acid iontophoresis. *Phys Ther.* 1992;72:133-137.

CHAPTER 10

"The Discussion": Time for Reflection

B ased on your process of analysis or inquiry, the discussion section suggests possible explanations for what happened in your case. It cannot offer bold statements of "conclusion," however. A case report provides insight into clinical practice through description and analysis; it does not provide proof of effectiveness.

Although the discussion is less structured than the case description, it should cover several topics. The discussion should provide the link to the purpose of the case report and to the literature, reflect on the case management and outcomes, suggest possible alternative explanations for what happened, and pose research questions. It may be tempting to merely summarize the case management and outcomes. Instead, invest the time and energy to thoughtfully reflect on what your case report *means*.

Link the Case to Its Purpose

A good way to begin the discussion is to use the first paragraph to remind the reader of the overall theme of the case and how your case is directly tied to that theme. In a case report involving a patient, the discussion usually begins with a general statement about the major clinical problem that the case illustrates, and it often includes a brief review of the patient's outcomes.

The purpose of the case report by Hahne and Ford[1(p1676)] was to describe the use of a functional restoration program for a patient with lumbar disk herniation associated with radiculopathy (LDHR). To link the case to its purpose, they introduced the discussion this way:

> This case report has shown how an FR (functional restoration) program supervised by a physical therapist was used to rehabilitate a 26-year-old female with a 1-year history of back symptoms and a 4-month history of worsening leg symptoms, with clinical and radiological evidence of an L5–S1 disk extrusion compressing the left S1 nerve root. Functional restoration has been shown to be an efficacious conservative management option for patients with subacute or chronic LBP,[32,33,35] but its effectiveness for LDHR (lumbar disk herniation with associated radiculopathy) disease is unclear.

In a case report by Rundell et al,[2(p88)] the purpose was to demonstrate the application of the World Health Organization (WHO) *International Classification of Functioning, Disability and Health* (ICF) to physical therapist management of 2 patients with chronic low back pain. The authors started the discussion by reflecting on this purpose:

> The WHO-ICF model is characterized by a bidirectional flow of information rather than hierarchical organization of its domains. This was demonstrated with several hypothesized bidirectional relationships in the 2 cases. The WHO-ICF model appears to provide an effective framework for physical therapists to better understand each person's experience with his or her disablement and assist in prioritizing treatment selection. It is notable that the health condition identified in this case series was LBP, which is a symptom-based condition rather than a specific, tissue-based pathology.[35] The WHO-ICF model assisted in identifying body structure and function deficits and activity limitations. Interventions directed at these impairments, contextual factors, and limitations addressed the health condition and appeared to affect activity and participation. For example, the hip muscle performance and length deficits observed in the patient with chronic LBP were hypothesized to result in poor segmental stabilization and consequent LBP. The WHO-ICF model may predict the potential success of physical therapy interventions for other symptom-based health conditions in which a specific, tissue-based pathology is unclear.

Neither of the examples above reviewed the patients' outcomes at the beginning of the discussion section, but a brief review often helps readers to grasp the big picture. An outcomes review is particularly helpful when the patient or patients had several outcomes or various outcomes over time. Schenkman and colleagues[3(p72)] reported multiple outcomes for 3 patients, which the authors then summarized in the discussion section:

> The 3 cases reported here also suggest that it is possible for people with mild or moderate PD to benefit from an endurance exercise program. Furthermore, the changes were not restricted to economy of movement, but extended to motor features of parkinsonism, physical functional capacity, balance, and flexibility. Perhaps most importantly, findings from these cases suggest that it may be possible to retain exercise benefits or even continue to improve for up to 1 year after a supervised exercise training program by performing home-based exercise with monthly follow-up to check on the adherence to the exercise program and performance of exercise and to provide encouragement.

Relate the Case to the Literature

As the discussion continues, it should provide evidence of how the case fits within the context of the literature. In the introduction section, you used the literature to identify what had already been done in your topic area and to identify the boundaries for your case; in the discussion, you'll focus on how your case and findings compare with what is cited in the literature.

In their introduction, Hahne and Ford[1(p1678)] cited literature on exercise-based rehabilitation for patients LDHR. The literature, however, was not conclusive, and the interventions often were not well described or standardized. To relate their patient management and outcomes to the literature, the authors wrote, in part:

> Consider how your case relates to a much broader knowledge base to help the profession bridge the gap between theory and practice.

> The patient described in the case report demonstrated marked improvement both clinically and radiologically. This report adds to the existing studies that showed favorable outcomes in patients with LDHR undergoing exercise-based intervention.[6,8] In those studies, however, patients may have also received epidural steroid injections, which have been shown to be effective as a stand-alone treatment,[3] whereas our patient did not receive such injections. Other case reports have focused on patients with acute LDHR for whom the prognosis was good[23–28] or on patients with chronic conditions without convincing clinical or radiological evidence of LDHR.[29–31] Several studies[11,17,19,20,22] have suggested that the majority of patients undergoing conservative treatment for LDHR demonstrate most improvement during the first 3 months following symptom onset, after which time surgery is often the recommended option.[1,2] Our patient had reported worsening radicular symptoms for 4 months prior to commencing her FR program, but she began to report substantial improvement 4 to 6 weeks after commencing the FR program. It is unlikely that resolution of the patient's disk extrusion commenced until her symptoms began to improve during her FR program, because studies[11,14,66] have shown that morphologic changes in disk herniations seen on imaging typically lag behind improvements in patients' symptoms.

Not all patient/client management proceeds as planned—and that's valuable to report. Moyers and Stoffel[4] started their discussion by commenting on their patient's unexpected substance abuse problem and then linked the problem to the literature to heighten readers' awareness of the extent of substance abuse on the job:

> This case required a pragmatic approach for working holistically to resolve an unanticipated problem of substance abuse that threatened the success of the client's rehabilitation plan and the outcome of returning her to work. Given that the incidence of dangerous substance use on the job ranges from 10% to 20% in the United States despite the existence of Employee Assistance Programs since the 1940s (Backer, 1987; Miller, 1995), the emergence of complications in rehabilitation related to a substance use disorder should not be surprising.

As you prepare to write your discussion, it is likely that you will go back to the literature to reread what you cited in the introduction and to seek other literature that may be helpful in explaining what happened in your case. Note how Vaughn and Nitsch[5(p1587)] placed their cases in the context of the literature:

Anatomical and hormonal differences also may have predisposed the patient toward developing a hypermobility dysfunction. Anatomically, females have less stability through the interlocking components of the SIJ compared with males. The joint surfaces between the sacrum and ilium are relatively smoother and smaller in females than in males.[78] The width of the upper facet occupies a third of the sacrum in females, whereas the upper facet in males occupies nearly one half of the sacrum.[78] Additionally, the joint surface in females extends only down to the upper border of the third sacral segment compared to the lower border of the third sacral segment in a males.[78] The hormones estrogen, progesterone, and relaxing fluctuate during the menstrual cycle.[79] There are conflicting research data on the effects of female hormones on ligament laxity. Although previous studies[79,80] showed a significant difference in anterior cruciate ligament laxity with increased levels of estrogen and progesterone, more-recent investigations[81–85] did not demonstrate a relationship between ligament laxity and hormonal changes during the menstrual cycle. The effects of hormonal changes on musculotendinous stiffness also have been investigated. Eiling et al[83] reported a significant decrease in musculotendinous stiffness as female hormones increased during menstruation. Although it was not known whether our patient's injury correlated with her menstrual cycle, a decrease in musculotendinous stiffness could have been related to the mechanism of injury.

Use the "funnel" approach

When relating your case to the literature, a "funnel" approach may help. First, think about the broadest dimension of your case, such as "manual therapy," "vestibular dysfunction," or "professional socialization." Even though your case may have focused on a specific application of a specific intervention, it is likely to be related to a much broader knowledge base in the profession. Consider how your specific case relates to this knowledge to help the profession bridge the gap between theory and practice. If your concrete example illustrates application of an abstract concept, make the connection explicit in the discussion. In a case report describing the use of locomotor training for a child with incomplete spinal cord injury, Prosser[6(pp1230-1231)] showed how theoretical models of neural plasticity can apply to a real patient. The discussion said in part:

Supraspinal changes in response to locomotor training support the belief that plasticity within existing neural circuits plays a role in recovery of function after locomotor training for SCI.[16,17] Activity-dependent plasticity within spinal circuitry also may play a role in behavioral response to training.[33,34] Neurophysiological function of the motor pathways does not fully mature until adolescence, and it involves increases in synaptic strength, conduction time, and effectiveness of temporal facilitation, as well as decreases in motor stimulation thresholds.[12–15] Little is known about the interaction between neuromaturational processes and training-induced plasticity in the nervous system. The effectiveness of locomotor training may depend on the maturity of existing locomotor networks. Although the child in this case was well below the age of maturity, outcomes did not significantly differ from those reported in adults.

She was, however, an independent ambulator prior to injury. The question remains whether locomotor training would be effective in infants or young toddlers who were not yet walking prior to injury.

In the discussion section of her case report of a child diagnosed with a sensory processing disorder, Dunbar[7] related the case back to Ayres' sensory integration theory. The information also could have been in the introduction to provide rationale for the testing and intervention. Dunbar wrote:

> A vestibular-bilateral and sequencing disorder is one example of the type of sensory integrative dysfunction a young child can experience. This disorder is characterized by poor postural mechanisms, inadequate bilateral integration, and underresponsive vestibular systems. Tests and clinical observations of Sara's difficulty with coordinating both sides of her body and her continuous movement in play indicated concerns in this area. It is believed that children with this type of disorder usually need more intense sensory input to perceive the same type of sensation as children without this disorder (Mailloux and Burke, 1997).

Whether your case lends support to or departs from the existing literature, you should continually monitor your language so that you do not slip into statements of cause and effect, such as: "In contrast to previous reports, I found that microcurrent electrical stimulation was very effective in reducing pain from peripheral neuropathy in patients with AIDS." You should state only what happened in your specific case, without making a claim that the intervention caused the outcome: "Although inconsistent with previous reports, the patient's lower-extremity pain decreased following microcurrent electrical stimulation."

Lowry et al[8(p700)] wrote carefully about the possible clinical application of an intervention approach for patients with patellofemoral pain syndrome. They did not imply any cause and effect:

> Although this case series cannot be used to show a cause-and-effect relationship between the manipulation techniques and the outcomes of the patients, the idea of affecting symptoms associated with PFPS through thrust and nonthrust manipulation of adjacent joints is intriguing and has been previously explored in the literature.[61,62]

Explain Your Hunches

Crow et al[9(pp1595-1596)] used their case to describe intervention for a patient with severely restricted hip motion following bilateral hip resurfacing arthroplasty. They posed another theoretical explanation for their intervention, careful to explain their hunches in the context of the case report:

> This intervention is intended to restore functional mobility and arthrokinematics of the severely restricted hip joint by improving the extensibility of the ligament-capsular tissue.[3,8,14,18,21,23-28] Furthermore, joint mobilization is intended to break up adhesions, realign collagen, decrease pain secondary to the stimulation of mechanoreceptors, and diminish muscle spasms and guarding due to nociceptive stimulation.[3,8,14,18,21,23-28] These mechanisms are all hypothetical, and there is a lack of evidence to date from basic and patient-oriented studies that can support these mechanisms convincingly.

Rundell et al[2] used broad theoretical concepts from the ICF to frame a patient case. In the introduction of the report, they used the concepts of body structures and functions, activities and participation, and personal and environmental factors; in the discussion section, they returned to these concepts as a central organizing framework for the discussion. Within the ICF framework, the authors explained their hunches about how a clinician can relate body structures and functions and personal and environmental factors to a patient's activity and participation. It's worth noting that this case report inspired dialogue on use of the ICF.[10]

Provide Alternative Explanations

Because case reports are not intended to prove effectiveness, the discussion section also needs to cover other possible factors related to the outcome. You know more about the case than anyone else does, and your well-reasoned alternative explanations can be important contributions to the professional literature.

Harris-Hayes et al[11(p210)] considered several possible explanations for their patient's improvement. Note that they used the discussion as an opportunity to "engage in a dialogue about the intervention"—not to demonstrate cause and effect:

Other factors may have contributed to the patient's outcomes. The effect of time on symptom resolution must be considered. Based on the time needed to achieve tissue healing, resolution of pain would be expected to occur within 4 to 6 weeks. The patient reported no noticeable decrease in her pain during the 3 months prior to her initial visit. She reported a decrease in the average intensity of her pain from 5/10 to 2/10 within the first week of physical therapy. So, it is unlikely that her symptom relief was due to time alone. The concurrent use of medications and ice may have provided the patient with relief of pain. She reported having used both Vioxx and ice during the month prior to her first visit and having experienced minimal relief. She discontinued the use of Vioxx before her second visit to physical therapy when she noticed a significant decrease in her pain. Therefore, it is unlikely that the resolution of pain was due to the anti-inflammatory effects of either the medication or the ice.

Sometimes the alternative explanation is not about possible causes of the outcome, but about *alternative patient/client management*, based on lessons learned. The discussion can be a time to admit "problems" and describe what effect the problems might have had, with suggestions for the future, such as: "[We] cannot determine whether these 3 individuals exercised at their target heart rates from months 5 to 16. Each patient was instructed in monitoring HR and in increasing speed or grade as necessary to stay in the target range. However, the 3 individuals were not adherent in recording their HR during each exercise session."[3(p74)]

Authors also have an opportunity to mention any missing or weak data. Harris-Hayes and colleagues[11(p211)] used a movement system impairment classification system in the diagnosis and management of a patient with knee pain; however, measures of tibiofemoral joint motion with estimated reliability and validity are not currently available. This was a limitation of the case, but it also made an excellent point about the kind of measure that is ultimately needed:

A limitation of this case report is the lack of specific criteria to indicate the patient's poor performance on the movement and alignment tests used in the examination. Clinical measures to determine rotation between the tibia and femur are challenging. Quantification of tibiofemoral joint motion is difficult, particularly when the patient is performing a motion such as walking. Despite these limitations, observational movement analysis is a key component of the physical therapy examination. We have established methods to standardize the test items; however, the reliability and validity of the methods have not been tested. We hope to develop future studies to address this deficiency.

"Where Do We Go From Here?"

The end of the discussion is a place to write about the direction that research should take. The case report provides an in-depth look at clinical practice, but it does not give definitive answers about what should be done with similar cases in the future. Statements from previous case reports ("Due to our small number of patients, the results of the associations reported in Table 5 should be interpreted with caution"[12(p1073)]; "this approach to treating children who demonstrate poor body awareness and who have a diagnosis of DCD does not appear to have been reported to date; however, caution is warranted about generalizing to other children with DCD because this case report concerns only one child and DCD is not a homogenous condition"[13(p465)]) indicate something about the nature of case reports: they should generate far more questions than answers.

> You'll generate more questions than answers

In the discussion of their case report on application of the ICF to 2 patients with low back pain, Rundell et al[2(p88)] made a comment that could be turned into more than one research question:

> Future research is necessary to apply the WHO-ICF model to other body regions and health conditions common in physical therapist practice. This research should establish the clinical effectiveness of its application and derive core sets that may be useful for optimal education, research, and reimbursement.

Because a major purpose of case reports is to generate hypotheses for future research to help answer important questions that clinicians are asking, editors and reviewers expect authors to include research suggestions in the discussion sections of their case reports. Cernak and colleagues[14(p95)] made a number of suggestions for future research in their case report on intervention for a child with severe cerebellar ataxia:

> Findings from this case report provide possible support for research demonstrating the importance of cerebellar structures in locomotor adaptation and in practice-dependent motor learning.[16,17] It also supports findings that the rate of locomotor adaptation and thus motor recovery may be slower in the presence of cerebellar pathology compared with other brain regions.[16,17] The intensity and duration of locomotor training using BWST required to achieve functional gains in patients with lesser severity of injury is not known. In addition, it is not clear how much additional therapy is needed to achieve these outcomes. Studies are needed to determine the optimal intensity and duration of locomotor training to optimize functional walking outcomes following cerebellar pathology.

Preparing for Peer Review

Just as peer review of clinical practice is intended to help clinicians as well as to ensure high-quality care, peer review of manuscripts is intended to help authors as well as to ensure high-quality articles.

Some components of the case report are best tackled after the main body of the paper—the "who, what, where, when, how, and why"—is done. That's because those components serve the function of "tying up the loose ends." They may be the finishing touches, but they're important. Because they actually serve as an aid to manuscript reviewers and editors, these details may help speed the review process. This manual uses *PTJ* and its review process to illustrate peer review; many of the points apply to other journals, but you will need to consult the author instructions for other journals that you may be considering.

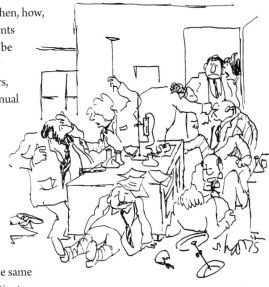

"IT STARTED WITH A SIMPLE CASE OF PEER-REVIEW."

Title and Abstract

The title of a case report tells readers at a glance what they should expect to learn from your report. The title should be as short as possible (ideally, no more 150 characters, including punctuation and spaces), while at the same time providing all of the pertinent information. If your patients are soccer players, for example, don't refer to them as "athletes" in the title; refer to them as "soccer players." For example, instead of referring to their patient as "athlete" in the title of their case report, Vaughn and Nitsch[1] were very specific: "female collegiate tennis player." As a reader, you know right away some important details about the main character in that story. Likewise, if the intervention you used was neuro-developmental treatment or strengthening exercises, say so; don't just say "physical therapy." The title of the case report by Nilsson et al[2] could have said "aerobic exercise in patients with chronic heart failure"; instead, it specified "group-based aerobic interval training...." Some other examples:

Vague Title:
Use of Motor Learning With a Child With a Developmental Disability

Improved Title:
Use of Random Practice to Teach a Child With Myelodysplasia to Transfer From Wheelchair to Car

Vague Title:
Rehabilitation for Glenohumeral Joint Subluxation

Improved Title:
Use of Functional Electrical Stimulation to Reduce Glenohumeral Subluxation in a Patient Following Stroke

Although the abstract is the first element in an article, it's better if you write it last; that way, you can summarize what you wrote in the manuscript, highlighting the most important details. Avoid such statements as, "Outcomes will be discussed." Give the important details. Don't treat them as though they are secrets to be revealed only to those who read the entire article! This does not mean that abstracts have to be long. *PTJ* will accept abstracts of no more than 275 words.

For examples of abstracts, look at case reports in recent issues of the journal to which you plan to submit your report. *PTJ* uses a structured abstract format, with topic headings clearly identified in boldface type. This not only helps readers quickly identify pertinent information, but helps you organize the abstract. For *PTJ*, regardless of the focus of the case report, abstract headings are: Background and Purpose, Case Description Outcomes, and Discussion.

Below is an example of a structured abstract from a multi-patient case report that had 4 purposes, published by de Bode and colleagues[3] in *PTJ*:

Background and Purpose: This case report describes the feasibility and efficacy of the use of constraint-induced movement therapy (CIMT) in 4 individuals (aged 12–22 years) who underwent cerebral hemispherectomy (age at time of surgery=4–10 years). The aims of this case series were: (1) to evaluate the feasibility of this therapeutic approach involving a shortened version of CIMT, (2) to examine improvements that occurred within the upper extremity of the hemiparetic side, (3) to investigate the feasibility of conducting brain imaging in individuals with depressed mental ages, and (4) to examine changes in the sensorimotor cortex following intervention.

Case Description: The patients received a shortened version of CIMT for 3 hours each day for a period of 10 days. In addition, a standard resting splint was used for the unimpaired hand for an 11-day period. Each patient was encouraged to wear the splint for 90% of his or her waking hours. The following outcome measures were used: the Actual Amount of Use Test (AAUT), the Box and Block Test (BBT), and the upper-extremity grasping and motor portions of the Fugl-Meyer Assessment of Motor Recovery (FM).

Outcomes: Immediately after therapy, improvements were found in AAUT and BBT scores, but no improvements were found in FM scores. Three patients underwent brain imaging before and after therapy and showed qualitative changes consistent with reorganization of sensorimotor cortical representations of both paretic and nonparetic hands in one isolated hemisphere.

Discussion: The findings suggest that CIMT may be a feasible method of rehabilitation in individuals with chronic hemiparesis, possibly leading to neuroplastic therapy–related changes in the brain.

Formatting Your References

The reference section immediately follows the discussion section. All sources of information cited in the text must be listed here. The rules of referencing are only slightly less complex than celestial navigation, but reference lists for case reports usually require knowing how to reference only journals and books and occasionally a Web site. The accuracy of a reference list can reflect well or poorly on the rest of the manuscript in the eyes of editors and reviewers, so it is worth spending some time to be sure it reflects well.

How many authors should be listed? Should you put references in numerical or alphabetical order? Should all the words of book titles be capitalized? Which bit of punctuation goes where? How do you abbreviate state names? The best way to find out is to look at the reference lists of articles published recently in the journal to which you are submitting your case report. Style manuals also can be excellent sources of information. The manuals that may be especially useful are the *American Medical Association Manual of Style*,[4] which is used by *PTJ* and many other health-related journals, and the *Publication Manual of the American Psychological Association*,[5] which is used by the American Journal of Occupational Therapy and other journals of interest to rehabilitation professionals. Instructions for authors sometimes specify the style that is used. Otherwise, just match your reference style to the samples provided by the journal articles—and remember to pay attention to all of those picky details!

Assembling Tables and Figures

When putting your manuscript together, place the tables, then the figures, after the reference list. As shown in **Chapters 7, 8, and 9**, tables and figures can be used to illustrate information that is difficult to describe or difficult for readers to grasp in text format. Tables and figures should not simply repeat information that is in the text; they should supplement the text.

> The rules of referencing are only slightly less complicated than celestial navigation.

TABLE 25. Hip Passive Range of Motion (ROM) and Normative Data[a,b]

Hip Motion	ROM, °, for:		X̄ (SD) Normative Hip ROM, °
	Left Hip	Right Hip	
Flexion	50[a]	110	118 (10)
Extension	5[a]	10	17 (7)
Abduction	20[a]	35	39 (13)
Adduction	5[a]	10	Not reported
Lateral (external) rotation	20[a]	30	27 (9)
Medial (internal) rotation	15[a]	25	31 (8)
Straight leg raise	30[a]	50	Not reported

[a] Empty (painful) end feel.

[b] Normative data derived from Roach KE, Miles TP. Normal hip and knee active range of motion: the relationship to age. Phys Ther. 1991;71:656–665.

Adapted from VanWye WR. Patient screening by a physical therapist for nonmusculoskeletal hip pain. Phys Ther. 2009;89:248-256; Table.

A usual way to incorporate tables or figures is to provide some background in the text, then refer the reader to the table or figure for the details.

Table titles and figure captions should give enough information so that readers can understand the tables or the figures without reading the text. This does not mean that titles and captions have to be a paragraph long! But they should include all of the pertinent details in a line or 2. One example of a table title: "Hip Passive Range of Motion (ROM) and Normative Data."[6] This title gives sufficient information to understand what the table is about without being too lengthy. As shown in Table 25, the labeling of elements within the table also can help explain the data. Any words that are abbreviated for the sake of space should be footnoted and spelled out at the bottom of the table.

Table titles typically appear above the table, and figure captions should be listed separately on a single page that precedes the figures in the manuscript. Instructions for authors, style manuals, and examples in journal articles are all sources of inspiration and information for creating tables and figures.

Submitting Video Clips

Today's journals are more than text. Today, along with their manuscripts, authors may submit video clips to show exactly what was done with a patient or an approach, as Chatham et al[7] did for their case report titled "Suspected Statin-Induced Respiratory Muscle Myopathy During Long-Term Inspiratory Muscle Training in a Patient With Diaphragmatic Paralysis" (Figure 40) and Schnall et al[8] for their case report titled "Gait Characteristics of a Soldier With a Traumatic Hip Disarticulation" (Figure 41). Both of these videos support the purposes of the reports and provide specific details that clinicians can use in managing patients and researchers can use in formulating clinical research questions.

Chapter 11: Preparing for Peer Review

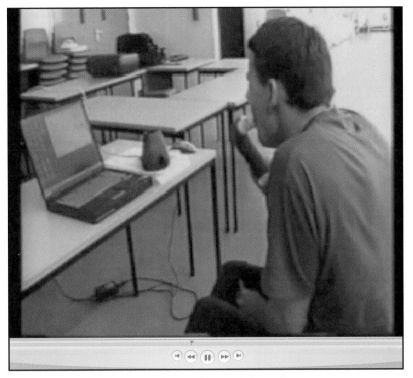

FIGURE 40. Still from "Inspiratory Muscle Training Video."

Available at: www.ptjournal. org/misc/videos/dtl. Chatham K, Gelder CM, Lines TA, Cahalin LP. Suspected statin-induced respiratory muscle myopathy during long-term inspiratory muscle training in a patient with diaphragmatic paralysis. *Phys Ther.* 2009;89:257-266.

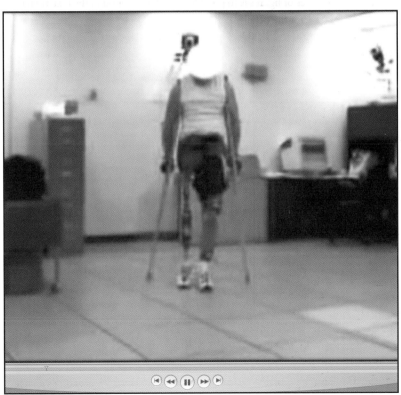

FIGURE 41. Still from "Gait Video of a Soldier With a Traumatic Hip Disarticulation."

Available at: www.ptjournal. org/misc/videos/dtl. Schnall BL, Baum BS, Andrews AM. Gait characteristics of a soldier with a traumatic hip disarticulation. *Phys Ther.* 2008;88:1568-1577.

In the case of *PTJ*, the entire review team reviews videos, unless masking would be compromised; in that case, the videos are either reviewed only by the editor or by the review team following acceptance of the manuscript.

You'll need to check with the specific journal to find out their technical requirements. *PTJ*'s preferred format for video clips is MPEG (Moving Picture Experts Group). Because of sophisticated compression techniques, MPEG files are much smaller than other formats for the same quality. These files are compatible with both Windows Media Player (PC) and QuickTime (Mac). Other acceptable formats include: .mov (QuickTime Movie), .wmv (Windows Media Video), .mp4, and .avi (Audio Video Interleave). Ideally, in terms of viewer ease, the video would be no more than 5 minutes in length. If the manuscript is accepted for publication, *PTJ* staff will convert the video file to MPEG format, and it will accompany the final print version of the article online. (For specifics regarding file size and dimensions, visit *PTJ* Online.)

Institute Your Own Review Process!

Once you've tied up all of the "loose ends," and before you submit your paper to a journal, ask colleagues to review your manuscript for you. They should be generally familiar with the concepts presented in the report, but they should not know the patient or be too familiar with your work. Be sure to tell them that you are not looking for praise, but that you want their help to identify every unclear word, weak transition, or omitted detail that the journal's reviewers are sure to notice. Remember: It's the praise of the reviewers that you want—not the praise of your friends.

While your colleagues are reading the manuscript, put your own copy away, and let it get "cold" for at least 2 weeks. Resist the overwhelming temptation to send the manuscript off as soon as it is finished! Fresh eyes will make problems much clearer, and you'd rather find those problems and fix them than leave them to the reviewers in whose hands the fate of your manuscript will lie. The final step before submitting the manuscript is to read the instructions for authors again to make sure you have included everything that is requested. If you are submitting your case report to *PTJ*, you can use the checklists in the **Appendixes** for your final "punch out."

Journal Peer Review: A Survival Guide

Although the mechanics of peer review vary somewhat among journals, the process usually is similar to that used by *PTJ*. The concept of peer review should be familiar to clinicians who have participated in both informal reviews (as part of everyday clinical practice) and formal reviews (as a component of quality improvement).

Just as peer review of clinical practice is intended to help clinicians as well as ensure high-quality care, peer review of manuscripts is intended to help authors as well as ensure high-quality articles. Manuscripts are not just "shot down" if they do not immediately meet publication standards. Editors work with authors to develop publishable manuscripts, using input from peer review. Understanding the review process used by *PTJ* (Figure 42) may help alleviate any anxiety that you have.

> It may help you to know that even manuscripts written by Editorial Board members— and the editor in chief— sometimes are rejected!

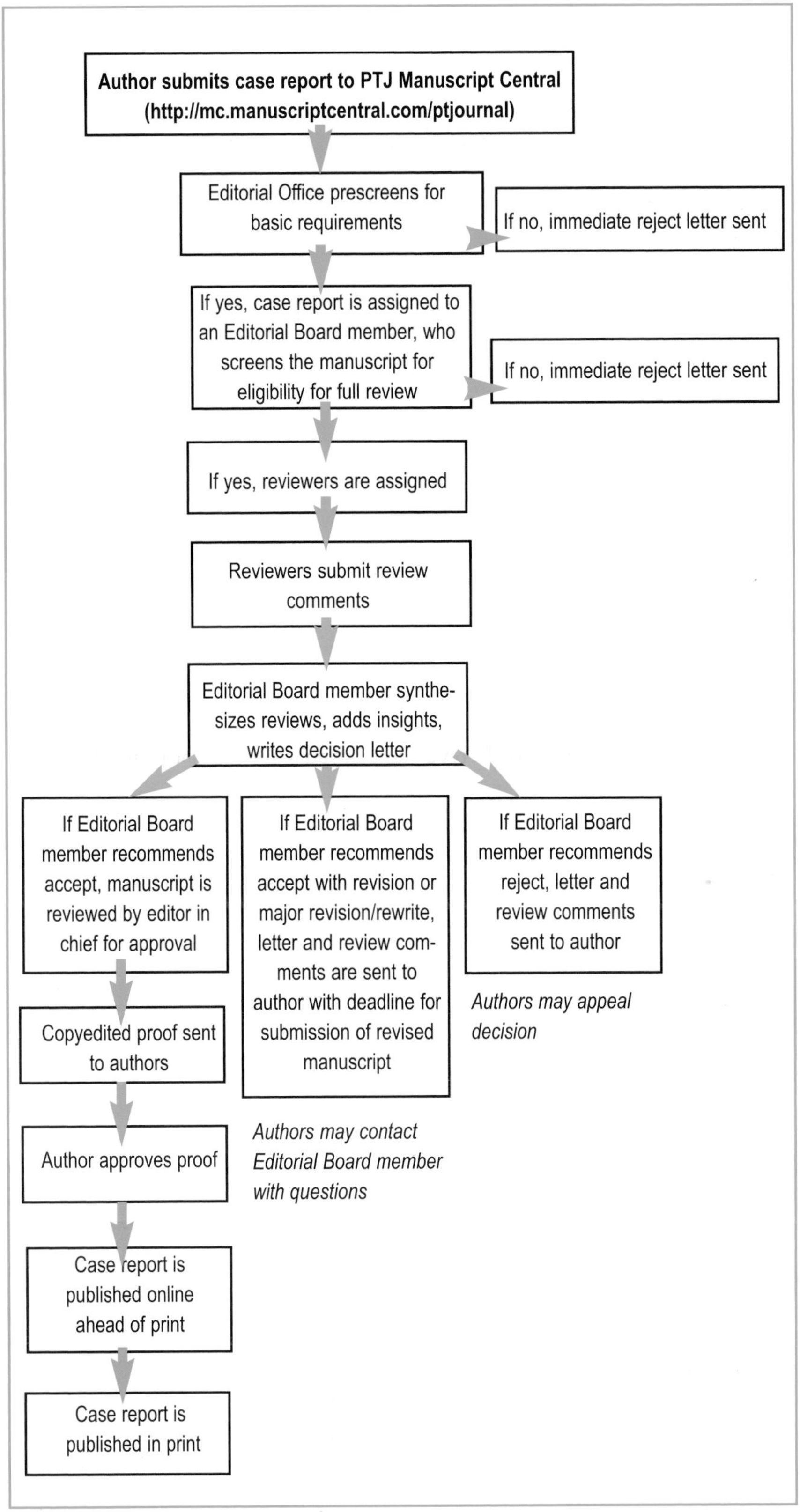

FIG 42. The peer-review process used by *PTJ* for case reports.

Author submits case report to PTJ Manuscript Central
(http://mc.manuscriptcentral.com/ptjournal)

Editorial Office prescreens for basic requirements

If no, immediate reject letter sent

If yes, case report is assigned to an Editorial Board member, who screens the manuscript for eligibility for full review

If no, immediate reject letter sent

If yes, reviewers are assigned

Reviewers submit review comments

Editorial Board member synthesizes reviews, adds insights, writes decision letter

If Editorial Board member recommends accept, manuscript is reviewed by editor in chief for approval

If Editorial Board member recommends accept with revision or major revision/rewrite, letter and review comments are sent to author with deadline for submission of revised manuscript

If Editorial Board member recommends reject, letter and review comments sent to author

Authors may appeal decision

Copyedited proof sent to authors

Authors may contact Editorial Board member with questions

Author approves proof

Case report is published online ahead of print

Case report is published in print

"What Happens When My Case Report Is Submitted to *PTJ*?"

Like all manuscripts, case reports must be submitted using *PTJ*'s online submission and peer-review system. The Editorial Office prescreens manuscripts to make sure that all of the necessary elements have been submitted and that minimal standards of readability are met. Manuscripts then are assigned to an Editorial Board member based on content area, and the Editorial Board member screens them for relevance and to ensure that the paper does not violate Journal policy (eg, prior publication). The manuscript is then assigned to at least 2 content-expert reviewers.

Case reports receive a masked review, which means that the identities of the author and the reviewers are not intentionally revealed to each other. The term "masked" is now used instead of "blind" because it is not always possible to completely conceal the identity of either the author or the reviewers, such as when authors cite their own previous work in the manuscript or reviewers make comments that only they are likely to make.

"What Do the Reviewers Do With My Case Report?"

The Reviewers carefully read the manuscript and:

1. **Highlight major strengths.** The reviewers briefly note what they believe to be the most positive features or important or compelling aspects of the report.

2. **Make major recommendations.** The reviewers assess the credibility of the case report. A credible case report convincingly explains why it makes an important contribution to the professional literature and how it relates to other literature. As described in detail in this manual, a credible case report also describes appropriate collection and interpretation of information, clearly explains the intervention, discusses implications for clinical practice, and proposes research questions or hypotheses for future research. Overall, it is the reviewer's job to comment on whether the case report has relevant content that makes a solid contribution to the field and has a clear relationship to existing knowledge. The reviewers also consider the organization and writing. A good case report is coherently written in a tone that is appropriate for the audience, uses correct and contemporary terms, and organizes the content into the appropriate sections.

3. **Make minor recommendations.** These comments may include specific suggestions for changes that could improve readability or comprehension but that are not critical to the credibility of the report.

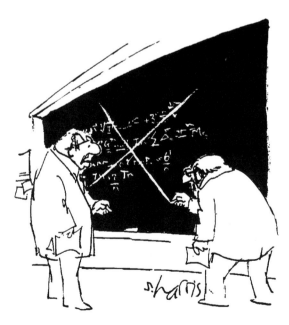

"That's it? That's peer review?"

The reviewers may make specific comments about specific sections, noting paragraph and line. They usually ask for clarification of anything that is unclear and offer suggestions for improvement. These comments are an excellent opportunity for the author to get input from peers with similar or greater expertise.

"What Does the Editorial Board Member Do With My Case Report?"

Once the reviewers have submitted their comments online, the Editorial Board member reads both the manuscript and the reviewers' comments. The Editorial Board member then synthesizes those comments for the author, adds his or her own insights, highlights what the Editorial Board member believes to be the most important issues, and guides the author when the reviewers disagree (as they sometimes do) about the manuscript. In most cases, the Editorial Board member will make the final decision regarding the manuscript; however, in some instances, a senior Editorial Board member will be consulted, and, in the case of accept recommendations, the editor in chief will review and approve the decision.

"When Will I Find Out the Results of the Initial Review?"

On average, the review of the first submission ranges from 45 to 60 days (like all journals, PTJ's goal is to continually shorten that time; note that in the previous edition of this manual, the estimated time was 3-5 months). In *PTJ*'s process, one of 4 possible decisions can be made:

Accept—No changes are required; *PTJ* staff will edit. This is a decision that even the most experienced and well-known writers have rarely seen on first submission and can only dream about! Revisions are almost always needed following first submission. If the Editorial Board member decides that the case report should be accepted with no further changes and the editor in chief agrees, the Editorial Office notifies the author.

Accept With Minor Revisions—The author needs to make minor to moderate changes before the case report can be accepted and copyedited for publication. This is good news. It means that no fatal flaws were detected during the review process and that, with some diligent attention to the comments of the Editorial Board member and the reviewers, the case report will be published.

Major Revision/Rewrite Before Decision. The author must make major revisions before a decision can be made. This category is used when there are questions that have to be answered and details that have to be provided before the credibility of the case report can be evaluated.

Reject—This usually means that the manuscript has fatal flaws and cannot be published. This decision also may be used when a paper has been resubmitted more than once but the authors have not responded adequately to reviewer concerns. If the authors believe that they can address the deficiencies, they always have the prerogative to rewrite the paper and submit it as a totally new manuscript, but this usually is not encouraged.

The Editorial Office sends the Editorial Board member's decision letter and the reviewers' comments to the author. Remember that the identity of the author remains masked from the Editorial Board member, but the author is given the Editorial Board member's e-mail address and is invited to communicate with the Editorial Board member about any questions. As hard as it might be to read some of the comments, the feedback can be a great learning opportunity, and, if the case report is eventually published, the process almost always results in a stronger article.

You might find it helpful to know that, just as there are stages of grieving, there are stages of dealing with feedback on manuscripts. As time passes, author reactions to the reviews range from "What? Those idiots were either too stupid to understand or too lazy to read what I wrote!" to "Well, I probably could have described that procedure more clearly," to "Some of these suggestions really are pretty good." The process takes time, and it is important to anticipate and recognize it so that you don't give up in that initial blur of anger, hurt feelings, and frustration that can occur in response to reading suggestions for improving your hard work.

In an Editor's Note titled "The Ugly Side of Peer Review," *PTJ* Editor-In-Chief Emeritus Jules Rothstein[9] offered some insight into the process and made some suggestions for how authors can direct their emotions in a positive way. He wrote, "Peer reviewers...become peer reviewers (for our Journal at least) only after they have been on the receiving end of the process, and most reviewers, including this Editor and the Editorial Board members, continue to publish and experience the process as recipients of reviews even as they review the works of others...." It may help you to know that even manuscripts written by Editorial Board members—and editors in chief—sometimes are rejected!

"How Can I Revise My Case Report Successfully?"

Your careful attention to the questions and suggestions of the initial review, indicated by appropriate revisions in the manuscript and explanations in a letter accompanying the revised manuscript, will help you avoid another round of reviews. To put things into perspective, the editors and Editorial Board members of most journals are volunteers, with busy personal and professional lives of their own. Their requests and suggestions are intended to maintain the journal's standards in the most efficient manner possible; every review means that they as well as the author will have less time to spend on other important activities! *PTJ* encourages authors to contact the Editorial Board member when they have questions about how to proceed with revisions.

"What Happens When I Resubmit My Case Report?"

Following the initial review, the Editorial Board member specifies who should review a revised manuscript—all or one of the reviewers of the first version, or only the Editorial Board member. This usually depends on the magnitude of the requested revisions. The review process for a revised case report is basically the same as the initial review process, except that this time the review team also is considering your accompanying letter that explains how you responded to their requests and why (or why you did not make the required revisions, if you disagreed with the requests). If the Editorial Board member decides that the manuscript needs further revision, the entire process may be repeated again. Most manuscripts need to be revised 2 or 3 times before a final publication decision can be made. If the Editorial Board member decides that the manuscript is ready to be accepted and the editor in chief agrees, the Editorial Office notifies the author. The time for review of a revised paper typically is shorter than the initial review.

"After My Case Report Is Accepted, Is That the End of the Process for Me?"

Not quite! Following acceptance of a manuscript, all journals copyedit to make the paper consistent with journal editorial style, and sometimes copyeditors insert "author queries" that ask the author to clarify any unclear language or to provide an additional detail based on final comments from an Editorial Board member. In *PTJ*'s case, authors receive a PDF of their edited article and are given the opportunity to review and approve or add changes.

Journals aren't just articles anymore—they're multimedia. If your case report describes an unusual challenge or a particularly insightful approach that relates to a larger professional issue, you just might be invited to take part in a podcast that accompanies your report! This is what happened to VanWye,[6] who published a case report on screening a patient for nonmusculoskeletal hip pain. His case report (and a case report by Chatham et al[7]) inspired a podcast discussion with VanWye and 2 noted experts in differential diagnosis and screening.[10] The participants addressed issues such as challenges in communicating with other members of the health care team, detection of red flags, scope of practice, and the physical therapist's responsibility to advocate for patients.

"How Long Does It Take to Get Published?"

Time from acceptance to publication varies widely among journals; however, many journals now release articles online ahead of print—sometimes by several months. Authors no longer have to wait for what seemed like forever to share their case reports with their profession!

The "Write" Stuff: Tips for Developing Writers

When going through school, most people who later become clinicians do not expect that they will also become authors. It's no wonder that many people who have wonderful cases to report are reluctant to try writing about them. *Tips for New Writers* (next page) contains some suggestions to help get you started, help keep you going—and help the product meet writing standards that may not be obvious to new writers.

TIPS FOR NEW WRITERS

■ If starting at the beginning is hard, start somewhere else. It's easiest to start with what you know best, which usually is the description of the patient or patients, what you observed, what you did, or what happened.

■ Don't worry about how the first draft sounds; just get something on paper. It's a whole lot easier to revise than it is to create.

■ Picture your reader as an advanced student or a colleague who is not in your area of practice. Although the reviewers and Editorial Board members will be familiar with the content area, they are responsible for ensuring that the report can be understood by a general rehabilitation audience. They will not read between the lines or make assumptions about missing information. Remember: It is much easier to take out unnecessary detail than it is to add details later.

■ Once you have revised the first draft—and second and third drafts!—let your manuscript sit in a quiet, dark place for a couple of weeks. While the manuscript is "resting," ask your friends and colleagues to read it and give you honest feedback. Give it to colleagues who know the topic—and to those who do not. A colleague who knows the area well can check for accuracy, whereas colleagues who are less familiar with the area are more likely to note omitted or unclear details. Then, with your own fresh eyes and your colleagues' comments, go through the entire manuscript again and make needed revisions. Send it off to your chosen journal only after at least the fourth revision!

■ Beware of unintentional plagiarism. Students and inexperienced writers often "half-copy" when they have trouble putting another author's flowing prose into their own words. Half-copying is what happens when you change a few words in a sentence or rearrange sentences within a paragraph, while retaining too much of the original source. Obviously some repetition of words and phrases from sources will occur (there are only so many ways of saying, for instance, that the quadriceps femoris muscle is a knee extensor), but if a paragraph follows the organization of a source paragraph closely and repeats a number of words and phrases, it should be rewritten. The easiest way to avoid unintentional plagiarism is to set aside the source articles after you've read them, and then write about what you gleaned from them.

■ Remember to use people-first terminology. Therapists work with people who have various conditions or problems, such as children with cerebral palsy (not "CP children") and people with brain injuries (not "the brain injured"). It is also important to refrain from using inaccurate, overly dramatic, or patronizing terminology, such as "stroke victim," "confined to a wheelchair," or "suffering from post-polio syndrome."

■ Use such terms as "functioning," "disability," and "activities," "participation," and "impairment" accurately. As discussed in Chapter 6, these terms have specific meanings as related to the *International Classification of Functioning, Disability and Health* (ICF) and should be used correctly to avoid any confusion on the part of the reader.

■ Use gender-neutral language, except when discussing a specific person or when sex is relevant. Avoid awkward and distracting terms such as "his/her" or "s/he." The easiest way to do this is to reword a sentence to use a plural pronoun or a neutral noun equivalent or to change the voice. For example:

Avoid: A therapist should observe how his/her patient moves.
Better: Therapists should observe how their patients move.

Avoid: The patient worked as a mailman.
Better: The patient worked as a mail carrier.

■ Avoid attempting to solve the gender problem by using pronouns that do not agree with the subject, such as "When a person [singular] has poor posture, they [plural] are at risk." This could be corrected in several ways. The easiest way is to use a plural subject ("When people have poor posture ...").

■ In general, make direct statements. One common problem: The identity of the performer of an action is obscured because the writer uses passive voice. In the active voice, the subject of the sentence performs the action of the verb.

Passive voice: The patient's knee range of motion was measured. (Who measured the patient's knee range of motion?)
Rewritten in active voice: The first author measured the patient's knee range of motion.

■ Resist the temptation to gratuitously scatter words that are meaningless, unnecessary, or imprecise. "Functional," for example, should refer to a specific function; "within functional limits," "functional activities," and "functional status" are all meaningless without clearly specifying the function to which they refer. Other examples of problem terms: "accurately measure" (why would you report inaccurate measurements?), "appropriately evaluate" (explain how you evaluated, and let the reader decide if it's appropriate), "clinically important" (is it important only to a clinician, or is it also important in the patient's life?), and "pain symptoms" (pain is a symptom).

■ Avoid ambiguous terms and jargon. Try to avoid ambiguous terms and phrases such as "tone," "strength," "moderate assistance," and "a home exercise program was given." If you decide that you must use them, provide operational definitions. That is, how did you define them for the purposes of this case report? Some jargon is so much a part of our professional language that we do not recognize it as jargon, or we protest that "everyone knows what it means." As emphasized in Chapter 4, everyone probably does not know what it means, or different people may have different notions of what it means. Clearly communicate what you intend.

■ Learn to be a better writer. Well-written manuscripts have a "professional" look in the reviewer's eyes (and you know the importance of an anticipatory set!). Many books about writing can be found in public libraries and are worth scanning. Many are surprisingly entertaining.

Suggested Readings

Day RA, Gastel B. How to Write and Publish a Scientific Paper. *6th ed. Westport, CT: Greenwood Press; 2006.*

Day RA. Scientific English: A Guide for Scientists and Other Professionals. *2nd ed. Phoenix, AZ: Oryx Press; 1995.*

Lamott A. Bird by Bird: Instructions on Writing and Life. *New York, NY: Anchor; 1995.*

Matthews JR, Matthews RW. Successful Scientific Writing. A Step-by-Step Guide for the Biological and Medical Sciences. *3rd ed. Cambridge, United Kingdom: Cambridge University Press; 2008.*

NEXT

It's Up to You!

Writing a case report is hard work, but it will be worth it. You'll gain insights into the process of defining, measuring, and describing for communication with the larger world. And perhaps putting words on paper will become less mysterious or intimidating. Who knows what doors you'll open?

References

1 Vaughn HT, Nitsch W. *Phys Ther*. Ilial anterior rotation hypermobility in a female collegiate tennis player. *Phys Ther*. 2008;88:1578-1590.

2 Nilsson BB, Hellesnes B, Westheim A, Risberg MA. Group-based aerobic interval training in patients with chronic heart failure: Norwegian Ullevaal Model. *Phys Ther*. 2008;88:523-535.

3 de Bode S, Fritz SL, Weir-Haynes K, Mathern GW. Constraint-induced movement therapy for individuals after cerebral hemispherectomy: a case series. *Phys Ther*. 2009;89:361-369.

4 Iverson C, Christiansen S, Flanagin A, et al, eds. *AMA Manual of Style*. 10th ed. New York, NY: Oxford University Press Inc; 2007.

5 *Publication Manual of the American Psychological Association*. 5th ed. Washington, DC: American Psychological Association; 2001.

6 VanWye WR. Patient screening by a physical therapist for nonmusculoskeletal hip pain. *Phys Ther*. 2009 Mar;89:248-256.

7 Chatham K, Gelder CM, Lines TA, Cahalin LP. Suspected statin-induced respiratory muscle myopathy during long-term inspiratory muscle training in a patient with diaphragmatic paralysis. *Phys Ther*. 2009 Mar;89(3):257-266.

8 Schnall BL, Baum BS, Andrews AM. Gait characteristics of a soldier with a traumatic hip disarticulation. *Phys Ther*. 2008;88:1568-1577.

9 Rothstein JM. The ugly side of peer review [editor's note]. *Phys Ther*. 1995;75:582-584.

10 Screening for medical problems and complications: where do we go from here? [Audio podcast]. *Phys Ther*. 2009;89. http://www.ptjournal.org/cgi/content/full/89/3/248/DC1. Accessed April 7, 2009.

PART 3

Appendixes

Appendix 1.

Checklist for Case Reports Focusing on Diagnosis/Prognosis

Emphasis is on the diagnostic or prognostic aspect of patient care. May cover the process and logic associated with differential diagnosis (ie, clinical decision making), unusual or difficult diagnostic/prognostic events, missed diagnoses, etc. Concentrate detail in patient history and physical examination and in conclusion or decisions made based on the examination. Challenge readers to deduce the diagnosis and to determine how the diagnosis relates to care of patient. May include interventions and outcomes, but detailed description is not expected there.

I. Title
- [ ] State that the manuscript is a case report.
- [ ] Maximum length = 150 characters (including punctuation and spaces)

II. Abstract
- [ ] Word limit = 275 words or fewer
- [ ] Structure: Background and Purpose, Case Description, Outcomes, Discussion
- [ ] State manuscript word count at end of abstract.

III. Body of Manuscript
- [ ] Manuscript word count = 3,500 words or fewer (excluding abstract and references)

A. Background and Purpose
- [ ] Provide scholarly discussion on the current issues related to the diagnostic/prognostic aspect of the case (eg, current state of knowledge, problems with differential diagnoses, mimicking or missed diagnoses).
- [ ] Provide rationale for why the diagnostic/prognostic approach needs to be demonstrated in a case.
- [ ] End with a purpose statement that clearly indicates the focus is related to diagnosis/prognosis (eg,"The purpose of this case report is to demonstrate the diagnostic process in … ").

B. Case Description: Patient History and Systems Review
- [ ] Provide detailed demographic characteristics and history (eg, chief complaints, other relevant medical history, prior or current services related to the current episode, comorbidities) to demonstrate that the patient is appropriate for the diagnostic/prognostic approach.
- [ ] Use relative dates (eg, years or months or days relative to onset of injury or to start of treatment) rather than absolute dates (ie, calendar dates). Reader will more easily grasp the chronology of events when the amount of time since the event or start of treatment is reported (don't force the reader to calculate the amount of time).
- [ ] Explain patient/family goals for physical therapy.

C. Clinical Impression #1
- [ ] Explain the primary problem.
- [ ] Describe the potential differential diagnoses.
- [ ] Identify additional information (not provided in the initial patient interview or history) that needed to be requested from the patient; explain how this additional information pertains to the diagnostic/prognostic aspect of the case.
- [ ] Describe the plan for the examination (eg, test selection).
- [ ] Explain why this particular patient is a good candidate for the purpose of the case report.

D. Examination

- [ ] Describe examination procedures that are consistent with clinical impression #1 and with the diagnostic/prognostic focus of the case.
- [ ] Clearly explain the rationale for using each test and measure.
- [ ] Describe the examination procedures so that others could replicate them; wherever possible, include figures, tables, and supplemental appendixes and videos.
- [ ] Cite available studies on reliability and validity of measurements. If not available, acknowledge this fact, and provide a presumptive argument for the potential of reliability and validity.
- [ ] Clearly explain all examination data.

E. Clinical Impression #2

- [ ] Provide a statement confirming or denying the initial impressions.
- [ ] Give a working diagnosis/prognosis.
- [ ] Indicate the plan of action (eg, proceed with intervention, further testing, referral for other consultation).
- [ ] State why the patient continues to be appropriate for the case. If the decision is to proceed to treatment, state the plan for intervention based on the current data.
- [ ] Include the plan for follow-up evaluation of outcomes (measures, time points). If further examination is required, address this next, indicating the additional tests and why particular tests are chosen.

F. Clinical Impression #3 *(optional)*

- [ ] If further examination was performed, state how the course of action was revised based on the additional information.

G. Intervention *(If the case report does not have an intervention associated with it, proceed to the outcomes section.)*

- [ ] Provide a general description of the physical therapy and/or medical/surgical interventions provided (eg, surgery, radiation therapy).
- [ ] Provide a general description of the intervention strategy, tactics, and procedures.
- [ ] Use tables, figures, and appendixes for the details, including only enough detail for reader to understand what was done; extensive details should not be necessary.
- [ ] Clearly link the intervention back to the diagnostic/prognostic decision-making process.

H. Outcome

- [ ] Briefly describe the outcome measures, and cite evidence for reliability and validity.
- [ ] If reliability and validity have not been estimated for a measure, acknowledge this, and make presumptive arguments that the measurements would be reasonably reliable and valid for the purpose of the case.
- [ ] Present the outcomes over the time points indicated in the follow-up plan above.
- [ ] Compare follow-up outcomes to baseline. Tables and figures can be used to enhance the description.

I. Discussion

- [ ] Provide a scholarly, critical analysis of how the diagnostic/prognostic dilemma—if any—was resolved, and how the process guided further decision making from a treatment and/or prognostic perspective.
- [ ] Compare the case to other relevant reports in the literature, and provide rationale for how this case makes a novel contribution and improves existing diagnostic/prognostic decision-making strategies.
- [ ] Offer suggestions for future research.

IV. References

- [ ] Cite no more than 30.

V. Tables and Figures

- [ ] Use no more than 6 tables and figures total.

Appendix 2.

Checklist for Case Reports Focusing on Intervention

Emphasis is on the intervention aspect of patient care. May cover the development of a new intervention or a modification to an existing intervention to deal with a clinical problem. Concentrate detail in the rationale for the new or modified intervention, the development process, the direct application to the patient, and the setting in which it is used. Remember that the patient history and examination should indicate why the patient is appropriate for the new or modified intervention. Include the outcome, but less detail is needed there.

I. Title
☐ State that the manuscript is a case report.
☐ Maximum length = 150 characters (including punctuation and spaces)

II. Abstract
☐ Word limit = 275 words or fewer
☐ Structure: Background and Purpose, Case Description, Outcomes, Discussion
☐ State manuscript word count at end of abstract.

III. Body of Manuscript
☐ Manuscript word count = 3,500 words or fewer (excluding abstract and references)

A. Background and Purpose
☐ Provide an underlying theoretical basis for the development of a new intervention or for the modification of an existing intervention.
☐ Provide a scholarly discussion on the gaps in the literature and in practice for treating the target problem, based on biological, physiological, biomechanical, psychosocial, or any other knowledge and theory.
☐ End with a purpose statement that clearly indicates the focus of the case as it relates to the intervention (eg, "The purpose of this case report is to describe the development and demonstrate the use of a new intervention for ….").

B. Case Description: Patient History and Systems Review
☐ Provide detailed demographic characteristics and history (eg, chief complaints, other relevant medical history, prior or current services related to the current episode, comorbidities) in sufficient detail to demonstrate that the patient is appropriate for the intervention.
☐ Use relative dates (eg, years or months or days relative to onset of injury or to start of treatment) rather than absolute dates (ie, calendar dates). Reader will more easily grasp the chronology of events when the amount of time since the event or start of treatment is reported (don't force the reader to calculate the amount of time).
☐ Explain patient/family goals for physical therapy.

C. Clinical Impression #1
☐ Explain why you believe that the patient is a good candidate for the intervention, based on the data collected thus far.
☐ Describe the plan for examination for further determining whether the patient is appropriate for this type of intervention (ruling in or ruling out relevant differential diagnoses, prognostic factors that suggest appropriateness for the intervention approach).

D. Examination
- [ ] Describe any tests needed to confirm that the patient is appropriate for the intervention as stated in the first clinical impression.
- [ ] Clearly explain all examination data.

E. Clinical Impression #2
- [ ] Discuss why the patient is appropriate for use of the target intervention, based on the examination data.
- [ ] Describe the plan for examination to determine the outcome of the intervention (measures to be used, follow-up time points), offering hypotheses about what should be observed if the intervention were to be successful.

F. Intervention
- [ ] Describe the intervention, including how the intervention was developed and how it was applied to the patient, in sufficient detail that others can replicate the procedure.
- [ ] May use tables, figures, and appendixes to enhance the detailed description.
- [ ] Provide the parameters of the intervention (ie, intensity, frequency, and duration) and rules for progression.
- [ ] State changes in treatment over time, along with the rationale for the changes.
- [ ] List any co-interventions that the patient may have received but that are not directly related to the purpose of the case; detailed descriptions may not be necessary.

G. Outcome
- [ ] If not already in the examination section, provide operational definitions of the outcome measures and their purpose, and cite evidence for reliability and validity. Priority is given to validated outcome measures. If reliability and validity have not been estimated for a measure, acknowledge this, and make presumptive arguments that the measurements would be reasonably reliable and valid for the purpose of the case.
- [ ] Present the outcomes over the time points indicated in the follow-up plan.
- [ ] Compare follow-up outcomes to baseline.
- [ ] Use tables and figures to enhance the description.

H. Discussion
- [ ] Reflect back on how the intervention may have assisted in addressing the target problem. This should be done in the context of other co-interventions that may have been provided. The key points of development and application should be tied back to the rationale for the treatment and literature on previous treatment approaches for a similar problem.
- [ ] Offer suggestions for further research.

IV. References
- [ ] Cite no more than 30.

V. Tables and Figures
- [ ] Use no more than 6 tables and figures total.

Appendix 3.

Checklist for Case Reports Focusing on
Application of Theory to Practice

Case demonstrates how a theoretical principle was used to develop an intervention, examination procedure, administrative/educational process, etc. Fully explain the theory, the implication of the theory for practice, and the development of an intervention or test procedure, etc, based on the principles of the theory. Supply detail about the patient or setting sufficient to show that the case is appropriate for demonstrating application of the theory. Outcomes may be reported, but with less emphasis.

I. Title
- [ ] State that the manuscript is a case report.
- [ ] Maximum length = 150 characters (including punctuation and spaces)

II. Abstract
- [ ] Word limit = 275 words or fewer
- [ ] Structure: Background and Purpose, Case Description, Outcomes, Discussion
- [ ] State manuscript word count at end of abstract.

III. Body of Manuscript
- [ ] Manuscript word count = 3,500 words or fewer (excluding abstract and references)

A. Background and Purpose
- [ ] Discuss thoroughly the theory to be demonstrated, citing the major references related to the theory.
- [ ] Discuss how you believe the theory could be applied to physical therapist practice, citing supporting literature; may relate to how the theory could be applied to an evaluation or intervention approach.
- [ ] End with a purpose statement that clearly indicates that the focus of the case is to demonstrate how the theory was applied to some aspect of physical therapist practice (eg, "The purpose of this case report is to demonstrate how [name of theory] was used to develop an intervention approach for....").

B. Case Description: Patient History and Systems Review
- [ ] Provide detailed demographic characteristics and history (eg, chief complaints, other relevant medical history, prior or current services related to the current episode, comorbidities) in sufficient detail to demonstrate that the patient is appropriate for the demonstration of theory to practice.
- [ ] Use relative dates (eg, years or months or days relative to onset of injury or to start of treatment) rather than absolute dates (ie, calendar dates). Reader will more easily grasp the chronology of events when the amount of time since the event or start of treatment is reported (don't force the reader to calculate the amount of time).
- [ ] Explain patient/family goals for physical therapy.

C. Clinical Impression #1
- [ ] Explain why you believe that the patient is a good candidate for the approach, based on the data collected thus far.
- [ ] Describe the plan for examination to further determine whether the patient is appropriate for this type of approach.

D. Examination

☐ Describe any tests needed to confirm that the patient is appropriate for the approach, as stated in the above clinical impression.

☐ Clearly explain all examination data.

☐ Provide a statement confirming that the patient is appropriate for the approach, based on the examination data.

E. Clinical Impression #2

☐ Discuss why the patient is appropriate for use of the approach based on the examination data.

☐ Describe the plan for examination to determine the outcome of the approach (measures to be used, follow-up time points), providing hypotheses of what should be observed if the approach were to be successful.

F. Approach

☐ Describe the approach (evaluation, intervention, or both) in detail. Details of how the approach was developed should be in the context of the theory being demonstrated. Descriptions of the approach should provide enough detail that readers can replicate them.

☐ May use tables, figures, and appendixes to enhance the detailed description.

☐ Provide the parameters of the approach (ie, intensity, frequency, and duration) and rules for progression.

☐ State changes in treatment over time, along with the rationale for the changes.

☐ List any co-interventions that the patient may have received but that are not directly related to the demonstration of the theory; detailed descriptions may not be necessary.

G. Outcome

☐ If not already in the examination section, provide operational definitions of the outcome measures and their purpose, and cite evidence for reliability and validity. Priority is given to validated outcome measures. If reliability and validity have not been estimated for a measure, acknowledge this, and make presumptive arguments that the measurements would be reasonably reliable and valid for the purpose of the case.

☐ Present the outcomes over the time points as indicated in the follow-up plan above.

☐ Compare follow-up outcomes to baseline.

☐ May use tables and figures to enhance the description.

H. Discussion

☐ Reflect back on how the approach adequately demonstrates the application of the theory to practice. The key points of development and application of the approach should be tied back to the original theory. Discuss whether the outcomes might suggest that the theory was successfully applied.

☐ Refer to previous literature to explain how it relates to application of this theory to practice as presented in the case.

☐ Offer suggestions for further research.

IV. References

☐ Use no more than 30.

V. Tables and Figures

☐ Use no more than 6 tables and figures total.

Appendix 4.

Checklist for Case Reports Focusing on
Clinical Measurement Procedures

Emphasis is on introducing a new clinical measurement procedure or modifying an existing procedure to deal with a specific problem or measurement topic. The difference between this category and diagnosis/prognosis is that the focus is on one specific procedure. Concentrate detail in the scientific rationale or theory for the procedure, the conditions under which the procedure should be used, and a thorough description of the procedure so that readers could replicate it (supplemental videos may be appropriate). The case demonstrates the clinical use of the test. If evidence of reliability or validity is not yet available in the literature, provide your own preliminary data, or make strong theoretical and presumptive arguments that the procedure provides reliable and valid measurements and has the potential to influence decision making.

I. Title
- [ ] States that the manuscript is a case report.
- [ ] Maximum length = 150 characters (including punctuation and spaces)

II. Abstract
- [ ] Word limit = 275 words or fewer
- [ ] Structure: Background and Purpose, Case Description, Outcomes, Discussion
- [ ] State manuscript word count at end of abstract.

III. Body of Manuscript
- [ ] Manuscript word count = 3,500 words or fewer (excluding abstract and references)

A. Background and Purpose
- [ ] Provide a scholarly discussion on the gaps in the literature for measurement of the target problem or clinical outcome that provides the rationale for either developing the new procedure or modifying an existing one.
- [ ] Provide the underlying theoretical basis for the development of the new test or modification. (This could be based on biological, physiological, biomechanical, psychosocial, measurement, or any other knowledge and theory.)

- [ ] End with a purpose statement clearly indicates that the focus relates to the clinical measurement procedure (eg, "The purpose of this case report is to demonstrate the use of a new clinical measurement procedure for....").

B. Case Description: Patient History and Review of Systems
- [ ] Provide detailed demographic characteristics and history (eg, chief complaints, other relevant medical history, prior or current services related to the current episode, comorbidities) demonstrate that the patient is appropriate for the target measurement procedure.
- [ ] Use relative dates (eg, years or months or days relative to onset of injury or to start of treatment) rather than absolute dates (ie, calendar dates). Reader will more easily grasp the chronology of events when the amount of time since the event or start of treatment is reported (don't force the reader to calculate the amount of time).

C. Clinical Impression #1
☐ Explain why the patient is a good candidate for the measurement procedure, based on the data collected thus far.
☐ Describe the plan for examination to further determine whether the patient is appropriate for this type of measurement procedure (ruling in or ruling out relevant differential diagnoses.)

D. Examination
☐ Describe tests needed to confirm that the patient is appropriate for the measurement procedure, as stated in clinical impression #1.
☐ Clearly explain all examination data.
☐ Provide a statement confirming that the patient is appropriate for the measurement procedure, based on the examination data.

E. Clinical Impression #2
☐ Describe how the results of the measurement procedure will influence decision making.

F. Measurement Procedure
☐ Describe the measurement procedure, including how the measure was developed and how it is applied to the patient, in sufficient detail that others can replicate the procedure.
☐ May use tables, figures, and appendixes to enhance the detailed description.
☐ List the basic rules and criteria used to interpret the results or scoring of the procedure.

G. Clinical Impression #3
☐ Present the results and interpretation of the measurement procedure.
☐ Describe how the results fit in with the other history and examination data to inform further decisions about interventions, referrals, etc.
☐ If the procedure results in intervention, describe the intervention plan.

H. Outcome (optional)
☐ If an intervention or consultation was performed based on the result of the measurement procedure, report the outcome of the intervention or consultation.
☐ Compare outcome measures to pretreatment measures.

I. Discussion
☐ Reflect back on how the measurement procedure helped identify the patient's problem(s) and assisted in treatment planning and evaluating clinical outcomes.
☐ Presumptive arguments might be introduced for the procedure's validity based on the case.
☐ Offer suggestions for further study of reliability, validity, and other measurement properties.

IV. References
☐ Cite no more than 30.

V. Tables and Figures
☐ Use no more than 6 tables and figures total.

Appendix 5.

Checklist for Case Reports Focusing on
Administrative/Educational Processes

Case describes or demonstrates the development and implementation of new administrative/educational processes or modifications to existing approaches to address special problems or needs. Detail is concentrated in the rationale for the new or modified process, steps taken to develop the process, and the direct application of the process in the context of the intended target population and setting in which it would be used.

I. Title
- [ ] States that the manuscript is a case report.
- [ ] Maximum length = 150 characters (including punctuation and spaces)

II. Abstract
- [ ] Word limit = 275 words or fewer
- [ ] Structure: Background and Purpose, Case Description, Outcomes, Discussion
- [ ] State manuscript word count at end of abstract.

III. Body of Manuscript
- [ ] Manuscript word count = 3,500 words or fewer (excluding abstract and references)

A. Background and Purpose
- [ ] Provide enough review of the literature to justify the development or demonstration of the process. Explain what has been done or not been done currently or in the past that justifies a change in the process or a modification of an existing process.
- [ ] End with a purpose statement that clearly indicates the focus of the case is to demonstrate an administrative/educational process (eg, "The purpose of this case report is to describe the development and demonstrate the implementation of an X management approach in outpatient physical therapy clinics to ....")

B. Case Description: Target Setting
- [ ] Provide details about the setting for which the process will be developed and in which it will be implemented.

- [ ] The description may include previous or current data about the setting sufficient to justify why this setting needs the process and why the facility is appropriate for it.
- [ ] State directly why this setting is appropriate for the demonstration of the process, based on the data provided in this section.
- [ ] Use relative dates (eg, years or months or days relative to start of event or process) rather than absolute dates (ie, calendar dates). It is usually easier to grasp the chronology of events when the amount of time since the event or start of the process is reported (don't force the reader to calculate the amount of time).

C. Development of the Process
- [ ] Provide a detailed description of the steps taken to develop the process.
- [ ] Support the rationale for each developmental step by the literature or other solid rationale.
- [ ] Discuss any other special considerations— such as, but not limited to, stakeholder consultations—that were taken into account in developing the process.
- [ ] Describe the plan to determine the outcome of implementing the process (measures, follow-up time points), providing hypotheses of what should be observed if the approach were to be successful.

D. Application of the Process

- [ ] Provide details of how the approach was implemented in the target setting
- [ ] Discuss the technical aspects of implementing the process, and identify the time-dependent factors (eg, frequency, duration).
- [ ] Describe any training procedures that were used for those involved in implementation of the process.
- [ ] Explain what was done to get acceptance by staff involved with implementing the process.

E. Outcome

- [ ] Discuss the outcomes of the actions taken to implement the process, consistent with the stated plan for determining outcome.
- [ ] Operationally define measurement procedures, if used.,
- [ ] Cite evidence for reliability or validity, if available. If such information is not available, acknowledge this, and make a presumptive argument.

F. Discussion

- [ ] Reflect back on how well the implementation of the process achieved its goals, based on the outcome data. Care must be taken to keep this discussion in the context of the case and not make generalized conclusions about use of the process in other settings.
- [ ] Discuss any difficulties encountered during the development and implementation of the process that could have affected the outcome.
- [ ] Refer to previous literature to explain how the application of the process in the case may or may not enhance administrative/educational processes in physical therapy.
- [ ] Provide suggestions for further research.

IV. References

- [ ] Use no more than 30.

V. Tables and Figures

- [ ] Use no more than 6 tables and figures total.

Appendix 6.

Checklist for Case Reports Focusing on Risk Management

Case describes risk management or demonstrates how risk management was handled. May cover such topics as accidents, adverse events, emergencies, and risk reduction strategies that are associated with physical therapist practice. Emphasis is on describing the nature of the risk, the rationale for dealing with the risk, methods for resolving or reducing the risk, and involvement of any other personnel or agencies.

I. Title
- [ ] States that the manuscript is a case report.
- [ ] Maximum length = 150 characters (including punctuation and spaces)

II. Abstract
- [ ] Word limit = 275 words or fewer
- [ ] Structure: Background and Purpose, Case Description, Outcomes, Discussion
- [ ] State manuscript word count at end of abstract.

III. Body of Manuscript
- [ ] Manuscript word count = 3,500 words or fewer (excluding abstract and references)

A. Background and Purpose
- [ ] Include a thorough review of the risk management topic (accidents, adverse events, emergencies), including the nature and prevalence of the problem and how it can affect physical therapist practice. Other consequences of the risks—such as legal, punitive, or budgetary and financial burdens—should be discussed to justify the importance of the topic.
- [ ] End with a purpose statement that clearly indicates the focus of the case is to demonstrate risk management in practice (eg, "The purpose of this case report is to describe an approach designed to prevent an adverse event X in the care of a patient with….").

B. Case Description: Details of the Risk Management Topic
- [ ] Detailed description of the patient involved (history, pertinent examination data, the plan of care, and any other events leading up to the risk management concern) or other entity.
- [ ] Discuss the current best-evidence guidelines (if they exist) to manage the risk and the expected consequences of deviating from the guidelines.
- [ ] Use relative dates (eg, years or months or days relative to start of event or process) rather than absolute dates (ie, calendar dates). It is usually easier to grasp the chronology of events when the amount of time since the event or start of the process is reported (don't force the reader to calculate the amount of time).

C. Clinical Impression
- [ ] Explain why you believe that the current situation represents the risk management issue.
- [ ] Describe what you believe needs to be done to correct, minimize, or prevent the risk at this point, and summarize the next course of action.
- [ ] Discuss plans for determining the outcome of the action plan.

D. Actions Taken to Address the Risk

☐ Describe in detail the actions taken to address the risk.

☐ Provide the rationale for the actions taken, using pertinent literature.

☐ If the actions involve the addition of an intervention, describe it in detail so that the reader can replicate it.

☐ If the actions involve interaction with other professionals, describe the purpose and nature of these interactions.

E. Outcome

☐ Discuss the results of the actions taken to address the risk, consistent with the stated plan for determining outcome.

☐ Operationally define measurement procedures, if used.

☐ Cite evidence for reliability or validity, if available. If such information is not available, acknowledge this, and make a presumptive argument.

F. Discussion

☐ Reflect back on how well the actions used adequately addressed the risk; take care to keep this discussion in the context of the case and not make generalized conclusions about how to address the risk.

☐ Provide suggestions for further research.

IV. References

☐ Use no more than 30.

V. Tables and Figures

☐ Use no more than 6 tables and figures total.

Appendix 7.

Checklist for "Full," Traditional Case Reports

Case describes the overall management of an unusual case or a condition that is infrequently encountered in practice or poorly described in the literature. The entire care of the patient—from start to finish—is described, with no one aspect of care receiving greater focus.

I. Title
- [ ] State that the manuscript is a case report.
- [ ] Maximum length = 150 characters (including punctuation and spaces)

II. Abstract
- [ ] Word limit = 275 words or fewer
- [ ] Structure: Background and Purpose, Case Description, Outcomes, Discussion
- [ ] State manuscript word count at end of abstract.

III. Body of Manuscript
- [ ] Manuscript word count = 3,500 words or fewer (excluding abstract and references)

A. Background and Purpose
- [ ] Provide a scholarly discussion of the importance of the topic, noting what has been published in the literature about the clinical problem and the key evaluation and treatment procedures.
- [ ] Provide rationale for why this case is needed.
- [ ] End with a purpose statement that is supported by the background information.

B. Case Description: Patient History and Systems Review
- [ ] Provide detailed demographic characteristics and history (eg, chief complaints, other relevant medical history, prior or current services related to the current episode, comorbidities) in sufficient detail to demonstrate that the patient is appropriate for the intervention.
- [ ] Use relative dates (eg, years or months or days relative to onset of injury or to start of treatment) rather than absolute dates (ie, calendar dates). Reader will more easily grasp the chronology of events when the amount of time since the event or start of treatment is reported (don't force the reader to calculate the amount of time).
- [ ] Explain patient/family goals for physical therapy.

C. Clinical Impression #1
- [ ] Explain the primary problem.
- [ ] Describe the potential differential diagnoses.
- [ ] Identify additional information (not provided in the initial patient interview or history) that needed to be requested from the patient; explain how this additional information pertains to the diagnostic/prognostic aspect of the case.
- [ ] Describe the plan for the examination (eg, test selection).
- [ ] Explain why this particular patient is a good candidate for a case report.

D. Examination
- [ ] Describe examination procedures that are consistent with clinical impression #1 and with the diagnostic/prognostic focus of the case.
- [ ] Clearly explain the rationale for using each test and measure.
- [ ] Describe the examination procedures so that others could replicate them; wherever possible, include figures, tables, and supplemental appendixes and videos.

- [ ] Cite available studies on reliability and validity of measurements. If not available, acknowledge this fact, and provide a presumptive argument for the potential of reliability and validity.
- [ ] Clearly explain all examination data.

E. Clinical Impression #2
- [ ] Provide a statement confirming or denying the initial impression, based on the examination data.
- [ ] Indicate the next plan of action (eg, proceed with intervention, further testing, referral for other consultation).
- [ ] State why the patient continues to be appropriate for the case.
- [ ] State the plan for intervention based on the current data, providing the plan for follow-up evaluation of outcomes (measures, time points).

F. Intervention
- [ ] Describe the intervention, including how the intervention was developed and how it was applied to the patient, in sufficient detail that others can replicate the procedure.
- [ ] May use tables, figures, and appendixes to enhance the detailed description.
- [ ] Provide the parameters of the intervention (ie, intensity, frequency, and duration) and rules for progression.
- [ ] State changes in treatment over time, along with the rationale for the changes.
- [ ] List any co-interventions that the patient may have received but that are not directly related to the purpose of the case; detailed descriptions may not be necessary.

G. Outcome
- [ ] If not already in the examination section, provide operational definitions of the outcome measures and their purpose, and cite evidence for reliability and validity. Priority is given to validated outcome measures. If reliability and validity have not been estimated for a measure, acknowledge this, and make presumptive arguments that the measurements would be reasonably reliable and valid for the purpose of the case.
- [ ] Present the outcomes over the time points indicated in the follow-up plan.
- [ ] Compare follow-up outcomes to baseline.
- [ ] Use tables and figures to enhance the description.

H. Discussion
- [ ] Reflect back on how the intervention may have assisted in addressing the target problem. This should be done in the context of other co-interventions that may have been provided. The key points of development and application should be tied back to the rationale for the treatment and literature on previous treatment approaches for a similar problem.
- [ ] Avoid any definitive cause-and-effect statements about interventions.
- [ ] Avoid making definitive generalizations to other patients.
- [ ] Speculate on potential implications for clinical practice.
- [ ] Offer suggestions for further research.

IV. References
- [ ] Cite no more than 30.

V. Tables and Figures
- [ ] Use no more than 6 tables and figures total.